THE WORLD AGAINST PANDEMIC

What's Next for Humanity?

HARISH ANKADALA

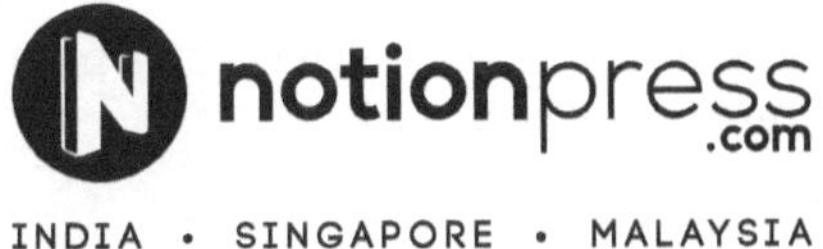

INDIA • SINGAPORE • MALAYSIA

Notion Press

No. 8, 3rd Cross Street,
CIT Colony, Mylapore,
Chennai, Tamil Nadu – 600 004

First Published by Notion Press 2021

ISBN 978-1-63714-551-7

Special thanks to:

1. Moses Misquitta
2. Shirin Joseph Vadakkan
3. Shanmukha Srinivas Naraparaju

CONTENTS

THE PANDEMIC

Hi, I'm Harish. I live in India, more precisely, in Mumbai. Some may have known Mumbai as Bombay. Yeah, I'm a Mumbaikar. A resident of Mumbai is called Mumbaikar in Marathi, where the suffix '-kar' means "resident of." It's not my birthplace, but I've been living here since my childhood. According to the United Nations' report (2018), Mumbai is the most populated city in the country and the seventh most populous city globally, with a population of approximately 20 million.

The seven islands that make up Mumbai have initially been the home of communities of the Marathi-speaking Koli people. For decades, the islands had been controlled by numerous native empires until they were ceded to the Portuguese Empire and finally to the East India Company when Charles II of England married Catherine of Braganza in 1661. Charles received the ports of Tangier and the Seven Bombay Islands as part of his dowry. It is now known as the financial capital of India. It is the wealthiest Indian city with a net worth of $950 billion, with 46,000 millionaires and 26 billionaires. It is also one of the world's top ten trading centres in terms of global financial traffic, producing 6.16 per cent of India's GDP and accounting for 25 per cent of industrial production and 70 per cent of Indian maritime trade (Mumbai Port Trust and JNPT).

You're never going to see Mumbai quiet. At night, the buzzing sound of the cars would make me believe that Mumbai never sleeps. I like to hang out at night on my bike with my friends, cruising quietly at 30 km/h while playing soothing music in my ears. Ok, I think it's the fantasy of most people. Mumbai is the most gorgeous at night. I don't know where you are, but if you're outside Mumbai, then you have to come and visit Mumbai, and if you're in Mumbai, then you have to see the most beautiful thing I've ever seen in the busy nights of Mumbai. If you've seen it and you're seeing it every day, then you're the luckiest person. One of the best ways to spend a good night in Mumbai is to take a stroll along the popular Carter Lane. It's a common destination for people to hang out with their loved ones, particularly during the night, when street lights illuminate and highlight the city's stunning view.

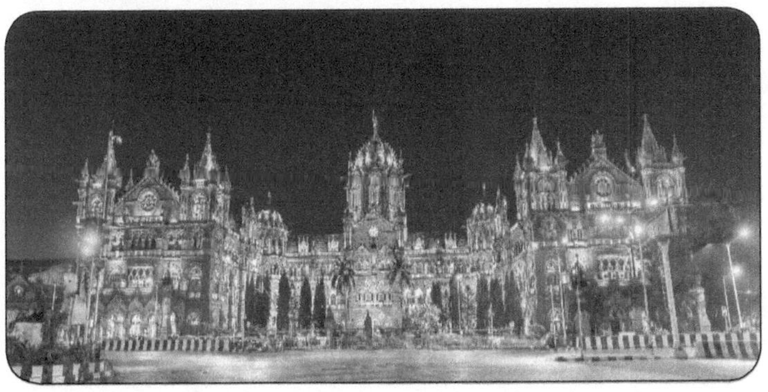

Trust me when I say this isn't New York. It is Mumbai. It's not just about the city; it's also about the slums in the city. Many might say, "Slums, so disgusting," but let me finish. Dharavi is a locality in Mumbai, Maharashtra, India. It ranks fifth in the world's largest slum and first in Asia's largest slums. It has an area of just over 2.1 square miles, with a population of around 1 million. It is one of the most densely populated regions of the world. It has a flourishing informal economy, with many slum residents employed by different household businesses such as leather, textiles and pottery. The total annual turnover is estimated at more than USD 1 billion.

Dharavi was an island with a prevalent mangrove marsh in the 18th century. It was a sparsely populated area. It was populated by Koli's fishermen before the late 19th century and was referred to as the village of Koliwada. Today, it is one of the world's most densely populated areas. Despite its high population density, it has a village feel and a central social square. 85 per cent of residents live in the slums and work locally, and some have also been millionaires. A lot of everyday activity is undertaken in the social sphere as people live next to each other. It helps to build a feeling of belonging. The aggregated literacy rate is 69 per cent. It sounds less, but with the tools they have and how they function, this number is enormous.

Mumbai is also known to have the most sophisticated transportation infrastructure in the country. Mumbai's public transport consists mainly of mass transit by exclusive urban rail lines, accompanied by main rail-lines servicing outlying suburbs, three local bus routes comprising the metropolitan city, public taxis, auto-rickshaws and ferry routes. The Mumbai Suburban Railway is the oldest railway in Asia, established in 1853. It is controlled by Western Railways and Central Railways divisions. The Government of India subsidizes the most economical transport through the Ministry of Railways. It has a length of 430 km and the world's highest passenger density as 7.5 million passengers travel in a day, which is more than half of Indian Railways' daily capacity. On a typical working day, boarding a train and going down are no less than baking cookies. On average, the suburban trains of Mumbai are only four minutes apart, leading to overcrowding. Mumbai trains carry passengers 2.6 times their capacity, making them the most crowded in the country. Bridges and platforms are under strain. Mumbai's suburban system carries 14-16 passengers per square metre of floor area. It ought to show how busy Mumbai is, but it's the best form of transport in terms of cost and time, and it's enjoyable too.

Mumbai is also home to six major religions: Hinduism, Islam, Buddhism, Jainism, Christianity and Sikhism. Hinduism is the most practised religion with 65.99 per cent and next comes Islam with 20.65 per cent followers, making Mumbai one of the most diverse cities. Mumbai's best feature is that most festivals are organized by groups of all religions and not just by a single community. A group can include people of all faiths. Like Diwali (Festival of Light), Holi (Festival of Colours) and Durga Puja are festivals that religiously belong to the Hindus but are celebrated by all, just like Eid, Christmas and other festivals.

This mixture of culture from religion, innovation, nightlife, classic old-world charm architecture, uniquely modern high altitudes cultural and conventional structures, and, most importantly, busy life surpasses Mumbai from any other city. I live in such a gorgeous place, and it's been 13 days since I stepped out of my house. In the next two days, I'm going out to pick up my groceries from the store for the next 15 days. Don't worry, I don't have agoraphobia. I'm a guy who isn't just going to stay at home; I enjoy hanging out with friends and family. I like getting fresh air and working out.

No festivities were recently celebrated. The mosques were deserted during Eid, and everyone celebrated Ganesh Chaturthi at home. The roads were silent, and the trains were not running. Don't worry, it's not the zombie apocalypse. But, because something has recently changed. Our Prime Minister, Narendra Modi, has called for a 21-day national lockdown from 24 March 2020. The lockdown was intended to be 21 days, but then it was extended by 15 days each time it was about to end. Officially, the lockdown concluded on 31 July. Post lockdown, public transit was not restored and offices were not opened. Many in the population were compelled to work from home. Actually, I enjoyed working from home. So what was the change? Why has the lockdown been applied for so long throughout our country?

It was the outbreak of the coronavirus that ceased all business, blocked all transportation and stopped tourism. Western railways had to bear a loss of INR 2,296 crore. Malls and shopping hubs had a loss of INR 1,00,000 crore. Theatres and films had a loss of around INR 1,000 crore. And it is just the tip of the iceberg. Some specific estimates state that the total loss is around ten times the loss that is estimated.

It's not just a tale of Mumbai, but it's going all over India, across the globe, for that matter. As defined by the traces of the virus, only eight countries were left uninfected. So, what's this virus, and what makes it so dangerous? Why do we have to follow the lockdown protocol? People claim it started in China, is it true?

Let me assure you that this is the best thing to start with, but not everything everybody thinks is true. I agree that I don't like China a lot, but it's because of the cheap goods. Don't worry. I'm going to prove a lot of hypotheses eventually. So, what's the outbreak and the pandemic? How is it influencing all the people? Will we have another pandemic, or have we had a pandemic in the past? How have we dealt with it?

It has been happening all over the world. Everyone in the world will relate to the word 'pandemic' and 'coronavirus.' It's been eight months since it all started, but we haven't found a cure or a vaccine for it. Why is it so challenging to create a drug or a vaccine for it?

Let's answer all the questions related to the coronavirus. But first, let's understand what is a virus and its anatomy? Let me take you to my next chapter, "Virus."

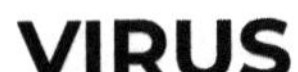
VIRUS

Life started on Earth at least 3.5 to 4 billion years ago and has been evolving ever since. Since the 19th century, scientists have recognized that any living being is made up of "cells." Cells are small bags of living matter that come in varying shapes and sizes. They were first discovered in the 17th century when Washington Teasdale invented the first modern microscope. Still, it took more than a century for everyone to understand that they were the foundation of all life. A few physicists have attempted to work out how early life could have evolved. They also attempted to replicate this Genesis moment in their labs to create brand-new life from scratch. Genesis deals with the beginning of life on earth. Unfortunately, no one has been successful. Many scientists are attempting to base their hypotheses on how life began on earth, and they have substantial evidence of their standing hypotheses. So, how did life start, and why is it so hard to make it? To understand this, we must travel to the beginning of the earth.

In the beginning, life did not evolve as a single cell. Creating a cell is halfway down the path of creating multicellular organisms. The process of creation of life on earth from non-living things is called abiogenesis. Everything in this world is made of atoms. Atoms are non-living things. When specific types of atoms came together to form a molecule and have a chain reaction with subsequent molecules, it led to some complex and self-sustaining chain reaction. This reaction was what made life possible on earth. Abiogenesis is a natural process by which life has arisen from non-living matter, such as simple organic compounds.

While the details of the process are still unknown, the prevailing scientific hypothesis is that the transition from non-living to living entities was not a single event. But an evolutionary process of increasing complexity, involving molecular self-replication, self-assembly, autocatalysis and the emergence of cell membranes. Although the occurrence of abiogenesis is uncontroversial among scientists, its possible mechanisms are poorly understood. There are several principles and hypotheses for how abiogenesis could have occurred.

The study of abiogenesis aims to determine how different chemical reactions led to starting a life on earth. It also determines that the weather conditions differed from what we have today. It's estimated that for the earth to have been the only case of hosting a technological species over the history of our galaxy, the odds of a habitable zone planet ever hosting a technological species must be less than 1.7×10^{-11} (about 1 in 60 billion). Life functions through the specialized chemistry of carbon and water and builds largely upon four key families of chemicals, i.e. lipids in cell membranes, carbohydrates like sugars and cellulose, amino acids for protein metabolism, and nucleic acids such as DNA and RNA. Any successful theory of abiogenesis must explain the origins and interactions of these classes of molecules.

Since life started on earth, we share our DNA and RNA with every organism on this planet. But the question arises, why do we share them? The answer lies in, how did we evolve? So, how did we evolve? Most importantly, why did we evolve? The first known single-celled organisms appeared on earth about 3.5 billion years ago, roughly a billion years after the earth was formed. More complex life forms took longer to evolve, with the first multicellular animals not appearing until about 600 million years ago. This evolution of life from unicellular microbes to multicellular life was pivotal in the history of biology on earth and has drastically reshaped the planet's ecology. Many theories are supporting how we evolved.

A collection of function-specific cells aggregated into a slug-like mass called a grex, which travelled as a multicellular body. This is one explanation for the origin of multicellularity. Essentially, that is what slime moulds do. Another theory is that nucleus differentiation was undergone by a primitive cell, thereby forming a coenocyte. A membrane will then form around each nucleus (and in areas occupied by cellular space and organelles), resulting in a community of connected cells in one organism (in Drosophila, this function is observable). A third assumption is that the daughter cells failed to differentiate as a single-cellular organism, resulting in a group of similar cells in one organism that might grow specialized tissues. That is what embryos of plants and animals, as well as colonial choanoflagellates, are doing. This hypothesis indicates that the first multicellular organisms, each with distinct functions, evolved from the symbiosis (cooperation) of different types of single-cell organisms. Over time, these organisms would become so dependent on each other that they would not survive independently, eventually incorporating their genomes into one multicellular organism. Each respective organism would become a separate lineage of differentiated cells within the newly created species. There are many more theories to prove how multicellular organisms started.

The first multicellular organisms did not have bones, shells or hard body parts, due to which there is no strong evidence preserved in the fossil records. One exception may be the demosponge, which may have left a chemical signature in ancient rocks. The Doushantuo Formation (a fossil Lagerstätte in Weng'an County, Guizhou Province, China) is noted for being one of the oldest beds to contain minutely preserved microfossils and phosphatic fossils. The microfossils and phosphatic fossils are so characteristic that they have given their name to "Doushantuo type preservation." The Doushantuo Formation has yielded 600 million-year-old microfossils with evidence of multicellular traits.

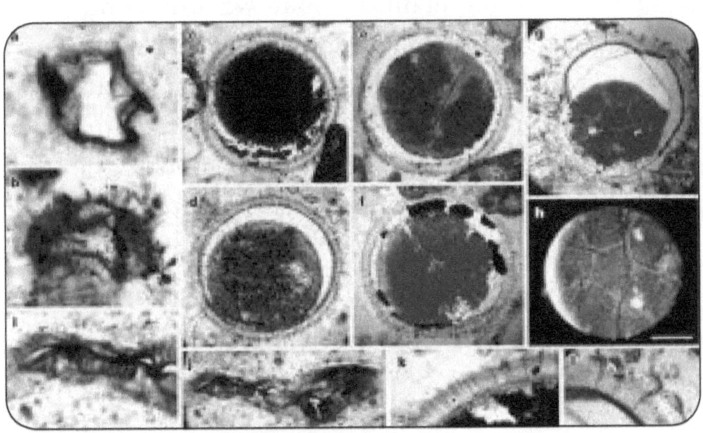

Evolution isn't a regulated mechanism. If it had been a regulated operation, we could have changed our bodies as we wished. Changing our body is an evolution too. But this is a partially managed operation. If you want to become dark, then you should lie under the sun. What's going to happen? Your body continues to make melanin to shield your body from sunburn. Melanin is a natural pigment on the skin. Hair, skin and eye colour in humans and animals depend primarily on their form and amount of melanin. It is produced by special skin cells called melanocytes. Everyone has the same number of melanocytes, but some make more melanin than others. People who have more melanin are darker than people who have less melanin. That's why Africans and Indians have more Melanin than Asians and Europeans do.

It's the evolution that has come in. If you're black, there's a 50 per cent chance that your next of kin will also be black. Only by exposing your skin to the sun for a long time can change your genetics. We cannot regulate evolution manually, but we can control the variables that affect evolution. This is the reason why the multicellular organism cannot return to a single-cell organism. As per history, evolution favours an individual with a higher probability of survival. But the question remains, why did nature not go back to a single cellular organism? There's an excellent explanation for that.

It's got everything to do with teamwork. Let me describe it to you. The cells benefited more from operating together than from living alone. They divided the workload among themselves, and, most noticeably, the body's lifespan increased. If a cell in a unicellular entity dies, then the entity is gone. But suppose a cell in a multicellular organism is dead. In that case, the cell may be replaced by cloning of the same segment, ensuring a multicellular organism's functioning and survival.

Fun fact: Every cell in our body replaces each other within seven years. It means we have a whole new body within seven years.

If you were a single unicellular entity, you'd die in 7 years, but now you'd survive for 60 years. You have 53 years to update yourself and share the same with the next generation. In nature, ants, termites, bees and so on exist in colonies. In reality, they behave as a single organism. Let me describe it to you. Every individual in a colony has a job to do. Let's take the ant colony, there are three types of ants. The queen (female ant that reproduces), the worker ants (perform everyday activities) and the male ants (fertilize female ants) function together as a single entity where each ant has a particular set of tasks to perform. If they weren't working together, then what are the odds of their survival? When they're together, they're battling rivals, they take care of the young and, most importantly, they share their bread. In fact, they have much-better maintained colonies in terms of planning and sustaining the structure.

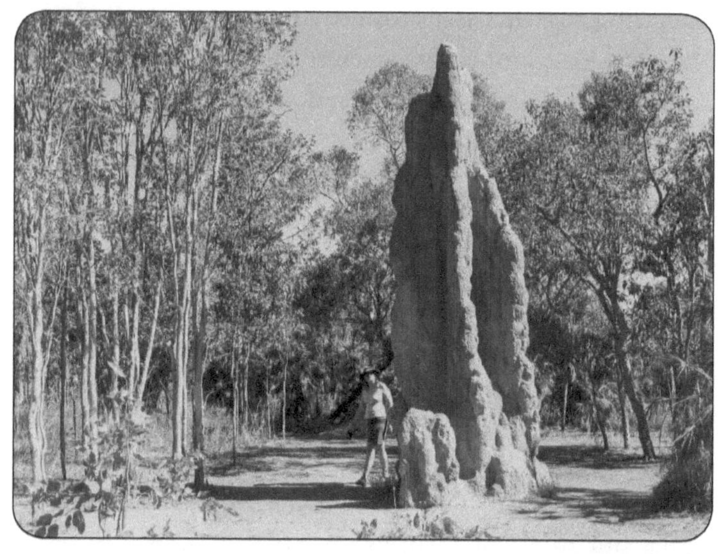

Everyone hates termites. Their total estimated damage to crops and human structures in the United States is $30,000 billion. Yet, there's one thing they are good at; they are good at building self-cooled structures. They show us how to build skyscrapers that are self-cooled. Termites in nature create skyscraper-like mounds that are ventilated by a dynamic tunnel system. The same technique was used by Zimbabwean architect Mick Pearce to render a natural cooling device by emulating termites' innovation. Termites may not be the most magnificent beings, but they build impressively tall dirt towers that can exceed 30 feet in height. If humans constructed a tower of proportional size, then it would beat the world's current tallest building, the Burj Khalifa, which is about 3,000 feet tall. Since coordination was the only way to guarantee the organism's survival, multicellular organisms did not revert to single cells.

They continued to grow into a variety of complex organisms.

One of the advantages of multicellular species is that multicellularity enables the organism to surpass the size limits usually imposed by diffusion. Single cells with increased size have a reduced surface-to-volume ratio and have trouble consuming and distributing adequate nutrients within the cell. Multicellular species have a strategic advantage of growing size with no limitation. Multicellularity also allows for increasing complexity by enabling the differentiation of cell types within a single organism. The vast majority of living organisms are single-celled, and even in terms of biomass, single-celled organisms are much more competitive than animals but not plants. Rather than seeing characteristics such as longer lifespans and greater size as an advantage, many biologists see them only as examples of diversity. But everything's got its flaws.

Our body is cloning our cells. It's a process, much like any other process. Cloning of a cell requires the transfer of genes, i.e. the much essential information, from one cell to another cell. In this process, anything can go wrong. When something does go wrong, the cell tends to kill itself, also called a failsafe mechanism. If the failsafe mechanism fails, the cells mutate uncontrollably. This is how cancer cells are formed. Cancer cells might also evolve when the standard control mechanism of the body stops functioning. Old cells do not die, instead expand out of control, becoming new, irregular cells. These extra cells may form a mass of tissue called a tumour. Multicellular species, particularly long-lived animals, face the threat of cancer. It typically happens as cells fail to control their growth within the standard development programme. Cancer is also defined as a loss of multicellularity in animals. There is a debate about the probability of cancer in other multicellular species. For example, plant galls have been characterized as cancers, although some scholars suggest that plants do not grow cancer.

Unlike animals, plants do not have a circulatory system capable of moving cells from one part of the body to another. If a cancer cell is deployed in our circulatory system, it will go to other body areas and establish a new colony. Again, this new colony is like cancer. It's the reason that when plants have cancer or tumours, they remain unaffected, but it's lethal to other organisms. As cancer is mutated cells that grow uncontrollably, they can also form a different form of cancer cells that can kill the host cancer cells. Cancer cells think of themselves as separate entities that live in other living things and feed on the host food source by linking them to the host veins. Similarly, as one cancer is developed over another cancer due to mutant cancer cells, the first cancer serves as a host. Cancer functions as an independent entity, which, in essence, extracts nutrients from its body, killing host cancer cells.

Since we have all evolved from a single cell organism, we all share some part of DNA. In humans, 99.99 per cent of DNA is identical. 99 per cent of our DNA is similar in primates, and 90 per cent of our DNA corresponds to cats. If we go below the evolutionary tree, the volume of identical DNA will begin to decrease but will ultimately reduce to 0.001 per cent. So, the virus or bacteria that we see in nature have the same DNA as we do. Yeah, that's the reason why we get sick. We can look into it later. Bacteria, which are very microscopic and single-cell organisms, share 98.5 per cent of genes. The human genome comprises billions of pieces of information and approximately 22,000 genes, but not all of them are, strictly speaking, human. Eight per cent of our DNA is made up of traces of ancient viruses. Another 40 per cent consist of repeated sequences of genetic letters, which are often considered to have a viral basis.

Being so similar and descendent, let's understand what viruses and bacteria are? Let's keep the fun for later and understand the bacteria first. What are bacteria? Bacteria are microscopic, single-celled organisms that exist in millions, in every environment, both inside and outside other organisms. Some bacteria are harmful but must serve a useful purpose. They support many forms of life, both plant and animal, and are used in industrial and medicinal processes. It is estimated that less than one per cent of the different types make people sick. Many are helpful. Some bacteria help to digest food, destroy disease-causing cells and give the body needed vitamins. Species commonly found in humans are Staphylococcus epidermidis and Staphylococcus aureus (potential pathogen).

It is one of the most natural microbes present in human skin and nose. According to the CDC, about 25 per cent of healthy people carry this bacteria. E. coli is a vital bacterial colonizer that our intestines require. We speculate that the ingestion of this particular molecule in leafy greens would be an essential factor in improving and preserving balanced gut bacteria and good digestive health. Research shows that leafy greens contain a specific form of sugar that contributes to healthy intestinal bacteria growth.

Almost all animal and plant life relies on the survival of the bacteria. Some microorganisms have the genes and enzymes required to synthesize vitamin B12, also known as cobalamin, and supply it via the food chain. Vitamin B12 is a water-soluble vitamin that is involved in every cell's metabolism in our body. It is a cofactor in the DNA synthesis of both fatty acid and amino acid metabolism. It is especially crucial in the proper functioning of the nervous system.

Baby koalas, or joeys, eat faeces from their mothers. They drink milk from a teat in their mom's pouch for the first six months or so, after they're born. The pap helps the baby develop and is full of intestinal bacteria from the mother, which may better prepare the joey for his adult eucalyptus-leaves diet. The presence of bacteria associated with Lonepinella koalarum, a microbe believed to digest tannins, is closely linked to health status. In most animals that depend on green foods, it can be observed. For their energy, termites rely primarily on cellulose within the wood. Wood has very minimal calories.

While termites feed on cellulose inside the wood, the wood is not digested by the termites themselves. Alternatively, microorganisms that live within the digestive system of the termite are called protozoans. These protozoans break down the wood inside the termite, producing by-products that both organisms can digest. It is a symbiotic relationship between the host and the organism. The host eats the food, and bacteria help in digesting food rather than wasting much of the host's energy and in turn the host gives them food and protection. If the bacteria stop working, then the host will die, in turn killing the bacteria. Thus, this symbiotic relation keeps both of them alive. In humans, gut bacteria are shared from the mother's milk and later some from the food we eat.

Bacteria also play a crucial function in agriculture. After certain crops such as rice or cotton are harvested or just about to be harvested, farmers also plant pulses and other grammes. These plants have bacteria in their roots that give nitrogen, also called atmospheric nitrogen fixation, which stimulates the plant's growth and provides them with sugars for their development. These bacteria can be present in the soil. Bacteria are essential in many phases of the nitrogen cycle. They recycle the nutrients by decomposition of dead bodies; the bacteria are responsible for this process's decomposition phase.

There are typically 40 million bacterial cells in a gram of soil and a million bacterial cells in a millilitre of fresh-water. There are approximately 5×10^{30} bacteria on earth, forming biomass that exceeds that of all plants and animals. If we were to lay all the bacteria one after the other, the bacteria's total length would be 2,64,25,020.8505 light-years. To put that in perspective, the distance between the sun and Pluto is only 4–6 light hours. You can do the math after that. Compared to bacteria, we are just a speck on the earth.

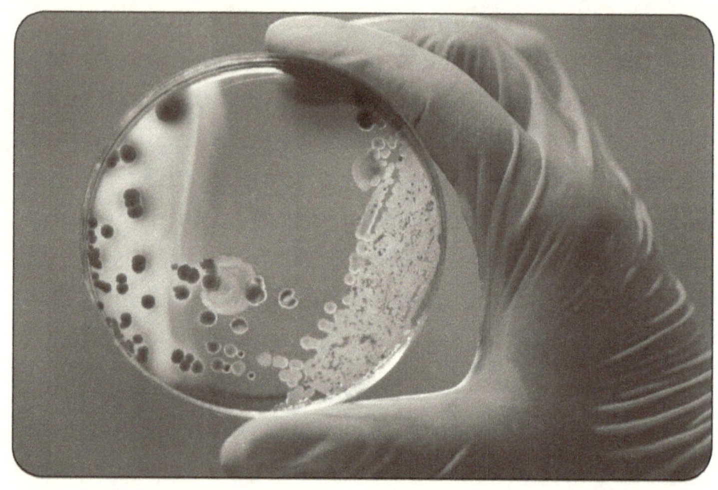

The structure of an organism defines a lot about it. A cell membrane surrounds the bacterial cell. This membrane encloses the cell's contents and acts as a barrier to hold nutrients, proteins and other essential components of the cell's cytoplasm, unlike eukaryotic cells. Eukaryotes are organisms whose cells have a nucleus enclosed within a nuclear envelope. Eukaryotes belong to the domain Eukaryota or Eukarya. They get their names from Greek word 'eu,' meaning 'well,' and 'karyon,' meaning 'nucleus.' They usually lack large membrane-bound structures in their cytoplasm. However, some bacteria have protein-bound organelles in the cytoplasm, which characterize aspects of bacterial metabolisms, such as the carboxysome.

Besides, bacteria have multiple components to control the cell division process. They lack the internal membrane since electron transfer reactions arise through the cell membrane between the cytoplasm and the periplasm. In certain photosynthetic bacteria, the plasma membrane is strongly folded and fills most cells with light-gathering membrane layers.

Some bacteria produce intracellular nutrient storage granules such as glycogen, polyphosphate, sulphur or polyhydroxyalkanoate. Bacteria such as blue-green photosynthetic algae, also known as cyanobacteria, create internal gas vacuoles, which they use to control their buoyancy, enabling them to travel up or down water layers with different light intensity and nutrient amounts. Not all bacteria are beneficial. Some are useful; others do not harm us. One per cent of the bacteria can harm us. So, how is it that they harm humans or some organisms? A bacterium that usually infects is considered a pathogen. They are the prime cause of human death from illness and infections—infections such as tetanus, typhoid, food-borne disease, leprosy, etc. In agriculture, the bacterial disease is also essential. They trigger leaf spots, mastitis, salmonella, anthrax in farm animals, etc. Yeah, the list keeps going on. The critical point is, how can they cause disease or infection?

The bacteria must first colonize the patient to cause an infection. When the host is invaded, they can replicate quickly. If the host is immune to the bacteria due to past infection or vaccination, then the host does not fall ill because the immune system can recognize the bacteria as a threat and eliminate them before they can do further damage to the body. Bacteria induce disease by secreting or excreting toxins, by internally generating toxins released as the bacteria disintegrate or by causing their antigenic properties to be responsive.

Bacterial toxins are proteins capable of conducting a variety of extraordinary activities. The toxin can be an organic matter or a non-organic molecule. They function as autonomous molecular machines, attacking individual cells in the body, punching holes in their membranes or altering intracellular components. The mechanisms of intoxication are incredibly dynamic. That's why physicists and physiologists are working on it to understand it better. Bacteria produce toxins that can be categorized as exotoxins or endotoxins. Exotoxins are produced and actively secreted. Endotoxins remain in the membrane of the bacteria. Endotoxins are typically part of the bacterial outer membrane, which is not released until the bacterium is dead. Toxins destroy enzymes and thereby compromise many of the body's functions that impede haemoglobin blood development, such as lowering the body's ability to resist free radical damage that accelerates ageing. Toxins displace structural minerals, resulting in thinner bones. As I said earlier, in order to potentially inflict damage, they need to multiply by millions. The question arises, how do they replicate so quickly?

Bacteria are single-celled organisms. They do not have male or female genitalia. So, they reproduce asexually. In asexual reproduction, the "parent" produces a genetically identical copy of itself. It is like cloning. They reproduce by binary fission and exchanging DNA.

Binary fission is a process in which fission itself means splitting. During the binary fission process, the parent cell copies its chromozone, forming two genetically identical copies. The cells enlarge and divide to form two daughter cells as they are a copy of the parent cells and are identical to each other too. This type of reproduction takes place very fast. Some types of bacteria can double the population in 10 minutes. This process makes it very easy to start their colony. So, how does the exchange of DNA take place since they don't have any sexual genitalia?

But not all bacteria are clones. They have DNA added from various places. It is how bacteria can acquire new DNA, and it takes place in three different ways:

Transfer of genetic material occurs during the process of bacterial conjugation. In this process, the DNA plasmid is transferred from one bacterium (the donor) of the mating pair to another (the recipient) through the pilus. The transition of DNA takes place during the wall-to-wall communication of the mating bacteria.

The bacterial transformation is a horizontal gene transfer process by which some bacteria take up foreign genetic material (naked DNA) from the environment. If the exogenous genetic material is identical to bacterial DNA, it may integrate into the chromosome. The bacterial transformation process deactivates most of the adverse effects of bacteria while retaining the same genetics from which antibiotics can be made.

Bacterial transduction is the process by which foreign DNA is introduced into a cell by a virus or viral vector. This can also be known as horizontal gene transfer as a viral transfer of DNA from one bacterium to another is its example. In this process of genetic recombination, the genes from a host cell are incorporated into the genome of a bacterial virus and then carried out to another host cell when a bacterial virus initiates another cycle of infection.

Being so aggressive, how can we kill bacteria? Antibiotics are effective medicines to combat bacterial infections. The word antibiotic means "against life." They kill the bacteria or stop them from reproducing, allowing the body's natural defences to eliminate them. The first modern antibiotics were used in 1936. By then, 30 per cent of the deaths were due to bacterial contamination. Antibiotics or antibacterials that entirely kill bacteria are called bacterial antibiotics. They attack the cell wall directly, causing damage to the cell. So they can no longer invade the body, preventing these cells from causing more damage. Other antibiotics block the growth or replication of bacteria called bacteriostatic antibiotics. They block nutrients from accessing the bacteria, which prevents them from separating and multiplying. Since millions of bacteria are needed to keep the disease running, these antibiotics will contain the infection until our body's immune system strikes.

Hence, any drug that destroys germs in your body is antibiotics. Penicillin is the most widely used antibiotic. Now, what are viruses? Can the use of antibiotics eliminate them?

Spoiler Alert:

Antibiotics cannot kill the infection caused by the virus. Antibiotics cannot kill viruses because they specifically attack the cell wall or the bacteria's reproduction organ. Since viruses do not have any of them, there is no target for antibiotics to attack. Antiviral drugs and vaccines can disrupt the reproductive cycle of the virus. To understand it better, we need to understand what a virus is?

The virus is a submicroscopic infectious agent that reproduces only within the living cells of the organism. Viruses infect all types of life, from animals and plants to microorganisms, including bacteria. A single virus particle is known as a vision and consists of a group of genes packaged inside a protective protein shell called a capsid. Some strains of the virus will have an extra membrane inside them; they will have an envelope. Therefore, the question arises, are the viruses really alive?

To keep things clear, we can think of them as zombies or werewolves. Are zombies alive? They are considered dead, but they move and perform some kind of function that's not productive. I'm waiting for the zombie apocalypse so that I can have my PPT prepared by one of them. Let me describe this to you in-depth. Not PPT and zombies, but viruses. They can also be compared to robots. How is that? Keep reading. So, how do we consider that something is alive? There are seven criteria to prove if something is alive.

Living things must maintain homoeostasis:

It's all about balance here. Can viruses regulate their internal temperature or its inner contents? Viruses aren't made of cells. The fundamental necessity is to be made up of cells. Viruses are organic matter, much like the organic matter used during the primordial stage of life. Viruses don't have nuclei, organelles or cytoplasms like cells, so they don't have a way to track or alter their internal environment. A single virus particle is known as a vision. It consists of a group of genes packaged inside a protective protein shell called a capsid. Some viruses have an extra protective membrane around them called an envelope. While the version should sustain a stable state, others suggested that the capsid and the envelope help virions survive changes in their environment. The conclusion is against life.

Living things have different levels of organisation:

Life is a complicated concept, and living beings represent the complexity of their structure. Smaller building blocks are coming together to make a larger product. Viruses are indeed doing this. They have chromosomes made from nucleic acids and a capsid made from smaller subunits called capsomers. So, the conclusion stands with life.

Living things grow:

Living things use energy and nutrients to become more extensive in size or more complex. Viruses, on the other hand, do not expand in length and cannot replicate themselves. They exploit the genes of the host to make a clone of themselves. While they pop out of the host cell, they pop out as a whole. So, they're not using their own energy or resources to reproduce. The conclusion seems to be against life.

Living things adapt to their environment:

Adaptation happens by unintended modifications that are beneficial to a whole population. However, they occur over time. They embrace a new environment and pass the genes on to the next generation. The virus will exist in two separate phases: the lytic process (where the virus replicates actively in the host cell) and the lysogenic process (where the viral DNA is inserted into the cell's DNA and multiples whenever the cell multiplies). If the host does not have enough resources or supplies to sustain the virus's replication, it will deliberately move to the lysogenic cycle. Where circumstances are right, the virus will gradually re-enter the lytic cycle. This skill is what makes the Human Immunodeficiency Virus or HIV. The virus begins to reproduce itself. This replication is what makes it so hard to destroy them. Medicine may destroy some viruses, but viruses that are genetically different or virus genomes absorbed into the host genes are left unaffected. The surviving virus will continue to infect other cells by making a copy of its strands. So, the virus cannot technically adapt to its environment by itself, even after being subjected to the environment for a long time. The conclusion stands against life.

Living things respond to stimuli:

It is one of the topics that scientists would debate about all day. It's one of the most contentious issues in the virus family. Response to stimulus is characterized by immediate external changes, such as the appearance of wrinkles in the hands when exposed to water for a long time or goosebumps when the unexpected, cool breeze touches. Mainly, no improvements were observed when the virus was exposed to touch, sound and light. As they feel nothing, the conclusion stands against life.

Living things use energy:

All the living things use energy, and they get energy from the food they eat. That energy is crucial for their survival.

Creating a new virion from scratch, including nucleic acid, and putting them together is a painful process and requires a lot of energy. All that energy that goes into production comes from the host. While they are being benefited from the energy, the metabolic process comes from the host. Technically, they do not have their source of energy, which can be used in its reproduction. It proves that they are just a bloth made up of organic matter and have the information needed to replicate only. The conclusion stands against life.

Living things reproduce:

One of the essential traits of life is to pass on genetic information to the next generation. The virus does multiply. A virus can multiply in thousands in a short period of time. But they must have a host to create more virion since viruses don't have organelles, nuclei or even ribosomes to replicate their genes. So, they hijack a living cell and use its tools to replicate itself, make new capsids and assemble everything. Technically, they are using tools from other living cells to replicate themselves as they cannot reproduce independently. They share genetic information with the living cell and manipulate it to replicate them. The conclusion stands against life.

An organism must qualify these seven characteristics to prove that it's alive. Out of the seven, viruses do not qualify in six traits. We should then proclaim that they are not alive, but they are organic matter, with a specific set of instructions that they appear to obey all the time. If the virus doesn't get the host cell to reproduce itself, then it's left to float in a vacuum. Viruses require a host to live and replicate, and most viruses can live for about a week without a host under the best possible conditions. If there are no hosts in outer space, then they can not live long. But the question arises, what happens if they interact with aliens? To answer this question, we need to understand how their genes interact and replicate?

We know that viruses cannot reproduce themselves. They need to hack the host cells and insert their DNA or RNA to replicate. Every cell has a cell wall, and every cell has a receptor. These receptors are like gatekeepers of the cell wall and only allow specific cells or particles to come in. Cellular receptors are proteins either inside or on the surface of a cell that receives a signal. In natural physiology, this is a molecular signal where the protein-ligand binds the protein's receptor. The ligand is a chemical messenger produced by a single cell, either by itself or by another cell. If the receptor does not meet the inbound receptor, the chemical can not reach the cell. That is why a particular form of the virus can infect only certain forms of cells.

That is also the reason why HIV is so dangerous as they attack our body's defence system, which makes us vulnerable to another disease. The immune system has many kinds of white blood cells to fight infections. HIV finds white blood cells, called CD4 cells. Your CD4 cell count gives you an indication of your immune system's health and your body's natural defence system against pathogens, infections and illnesses. CD4 cells are sometimes also called T-cells, T-lymphocytes or helper cells. These receptor cells are the first line of defence. There are two possibilities in this case. Some viruses only put in their replicating genes, including the virus's DNA and other build material, and some viruses go inside the cell. They are a fraction of the size of a cell or most of the bacteria.

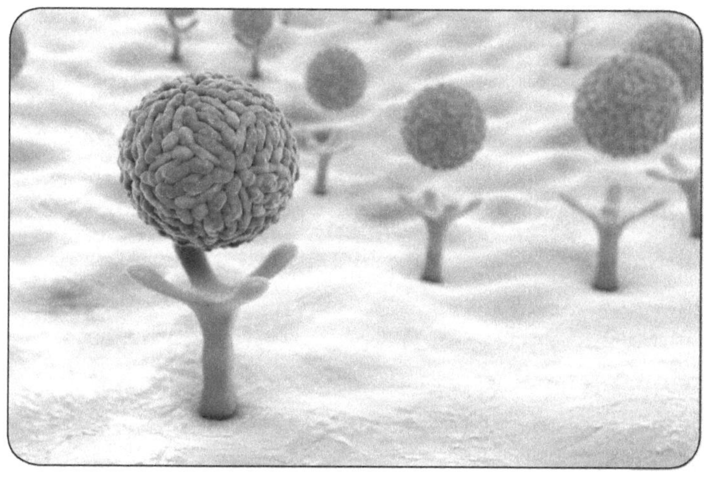

The above image shows a chemical binding with a receptor of another cell. This image is just a graphical depiction.

When within the cell, the viral capsid is dissolved and degraded by viral enzymes or host enzymes that produce viral genomic nucleic acid. The replication process is complex, and this process often varies whether the virus is made up of DNA or RNA. There are also two types of DNA viruses: single-stranded and double-stranded. Many double-stranded DNA viruses replicate inside the host cell nucleus, namely polyomaviruses, adenoviruses and herpesviruses. A lot of experiments are ongoing for single-stranded viruses. However, we do not have many hypotheses to describe how humans or other species are influenced. However, they also impact vertebrates, organs with a spinal cord surrounded by cartilage or bone. Two examples are circoviridae and parvoviridae. They reproduce inside the nucleus and form a double-stranded intermediate DNA during replication.

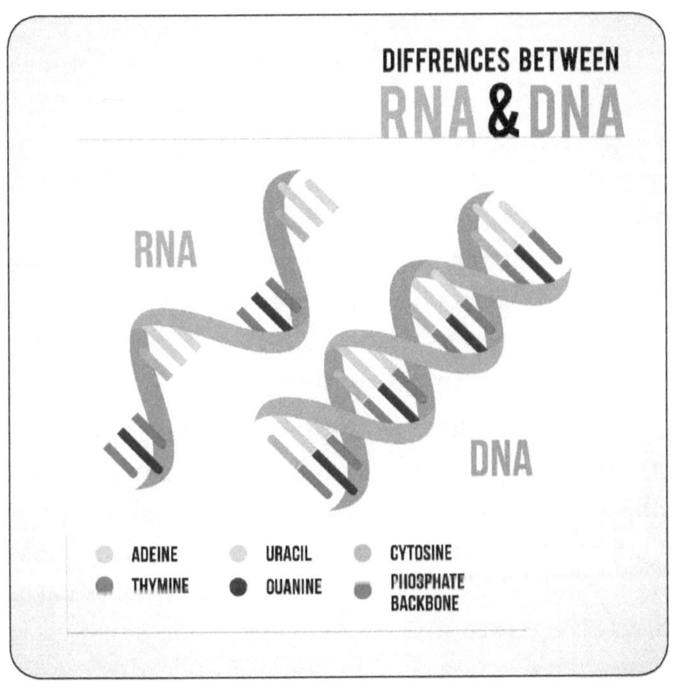

The above graphical image shows the difference between RNA and DNA.

RNA replicating viruses also have two forms: single-stranded and double-stranded. A lot of experiments are ongoing on the double-stranded RNA virus. In this process, the host RNA is connected to the virus RNA. Apart from the virus RNA, double-stranded RNA virus binds itself to the host RNA and then replicates itself.

The single-stranded mechanism is the same, but the distinction is that single-stranded RNA is made in this case. The process of replication culminates in the de novo synthesis of viral proteins and genomes. When they've replicated themselves, they're starting to assemble and get ready to release the virus.

De novo synthesis of the viral genome and proteins that are post-transcriptionally modified. In molecular biology and genetics, transcriptional regulation is how the cell controls the transfer of DNA to RNA. Once the virus genome is modified, viral proteins are packaged with the newly replicated viral genome into new virions are ready for release from the host cell. This mechanism is also referred to as maturation. The release process is much more interesting than that.

This process has two types. Cytolytic (cytolysis, or osmotic lysis) occurs when a cell bursts due to an osmotic imbalance that has caused excess water to diffuse into the cell, leading to the death of the cell. The other method is cytopathic viruses (cytopathic effect or cytopathogenic effect). It refers to structural changes in host cells caused by the viral invasion. It does not lead to death.

In the cytolytic phase, the cell dies because of its insufficient resources. In certain instances, where the cell explodes as the virus tries to get out of the cell, the cell can die. The best example of this is Variola Major, also known as smallpox. Cytopathic viruses, such as influenza A virus, are usually released from the host cell by budding. Budding is a form of asexual reproduction in which a new organism grows from an outgrowth or bud due to cell division at a specific site. So, in this situation, it seems like they're reproducing, but it's just the virus that comes out of the cell. It is this mechanism that results in the acquisition of a viral phospholipid envelope. Since the virus comes out of the host cell, several viral proteins remain inside the host cell membrane, serving as other possible targets. Viral DNA or RNA is integrated into the DNA of the cells. Viral DNA is, therefore, multiplied as the cell reproduces. After any physical or chemical mutation, the DNA virus will activate and budge out of the cell or occasionally it will merely blast out of the cell.

In some instances, this mechanism can also destroy the host cell. Owing to this accelerated mutation of the virus, it is complicated to kill the virus. Often a medicine that kills a virus cannot kill the same mutated virus. However, the odds of replicating them are still pretty low and so are the chances of killing them. Unlike bacteria, viruses do not have a cell wall that has broken the chance of survival. Being so immune to drugs, it's hard to kill them. It is why we can cure the symptoms of the cold, but not the cold itself. Since the common cold comprises hundreds of various types of viruses, it is challenging to make antiviral drugs for viruses and mutated viruses. So, the best way to approach it is by treating the symptoms to control the situation. We cannot tell what number of viruses are dangerous to us. In reality, many viruses are useful as they are used to kill bacteria. Phage therapy is the therapeutic use of viruses to treat pathogenic bacterial infections. Bacteriophages, known as phages, are a form of viruses. Since there are no specific medicines to kill a virus, it all depends on our immune system. Let's get into it later.

Answering the question of what would happen if a virus comes into contact with an alien? Since the virus uses the host's resources to replicate itself, aliens must also have the same building materials. Viruses are known to jump from species to species. But most of the time, they are unsuccessful. We will see more about it in "everything comes from somewhere." First of all, they must all have the same DNA or RNA. What are the odds of having it? The chances of the existence of life on earth are 1.7×10^{-11} (about 1 in 60 billion). The chances of the existence of earth are 1 in 700 quintillions. What are the chances that some planet in the universe has the same probability of existence and the same possibility of having a life form?

Well, I am a science student. I would say the chances are next to zero but not zero. If they have the same morphology as us, they will also react to the virus-like us, unless their bodies are resilient. Yes, that is also a possibility, or they might have genes that are not as developed as us and might get affected due to the virus, which can also lead to the extension of the species. Keeping aliens aside, if a virus moves from dogs to humans, the virus might not even survive. It will be like they have moved to another planet. A virus can rarely mutate, hit the jackpot and jump from species. Jumping into an alien species feels impossible but not impossible.

What if they have different building materials? If they don't have the building materials needed for the virus to replicate, the virus might go extinct. It would have been the story of the past. They might also not have the option to mutate, since the building blocks are different. Viruses are coded to use certain types of chemicals to make the materials needed to build itself. Without those materials, the virus cannot replicate, and they might die. The possibilities are endless, and no one can predict the future. If a virus that comes from outer space infects us, the odds of survival are high. But there are chances that we could get infected or, in most likely cases, go extinct.

So, will this coronavirus lead to an extinction or mass death? Well, you will have to wait until the end to know that. Before we understand that, we need to know how our body protects us from harmful viruses and bacteria? Let me take you to my next chapter, "Our Immune System."

OUR IMMUNE SYSTEM

It may not sound like much, but our immune system is probably one of the most important reasons we live. Researchers are still working on understanding how our body fights any incoming threats, including a virus. The immune system is a complex network of cells and proteins that defends the body against infection. It keeps a record of every germ (microbe) it has ever defeated to recognize and destroy the microbe quickly if it enters the body again. But how do they know if a particular cell or an incoming microbe is a germ, and most importantly, how do they kill it?

Spoiler Alert: Our body continuously plays a lottery with us. It is a good thing. Let me explain it to you.

Our immune system consists of seven parts. They are thymus, bone marrow, spleen, antibiotics, white blood cells, the complement system and the lymphatic system.

Thymus: It is a specialized primary lymphoid organ of the immune system. Within it, Thymus cell lymphocytes (T cells) mature. T cells are critical to the adaptive immune system, where the body adapts specifically to foreign invaders.

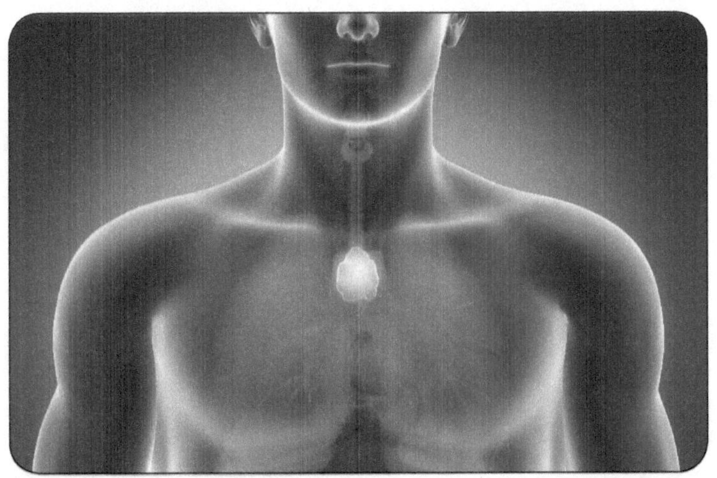

Thymus filters and monitors your blood content and also produces white blood cells. It starts deteriorating after birth, but the process speeds up after puberty. And by age 65, we are unable to make new T-cells. As the organ shrinks, the T-cell areas are replaced with fatty tissue in a process called involution. It is the reason you are vulnerable to more disease once you grow old.

Bone marrow: It is the soft spongy tissue inside the bone that makes blood. Blood cells include white blood, red blood and platelets. White blood helps us fight infections; red blood helps us carry oxygen throughout the body, and platelets help us clot blood when it bleeds.

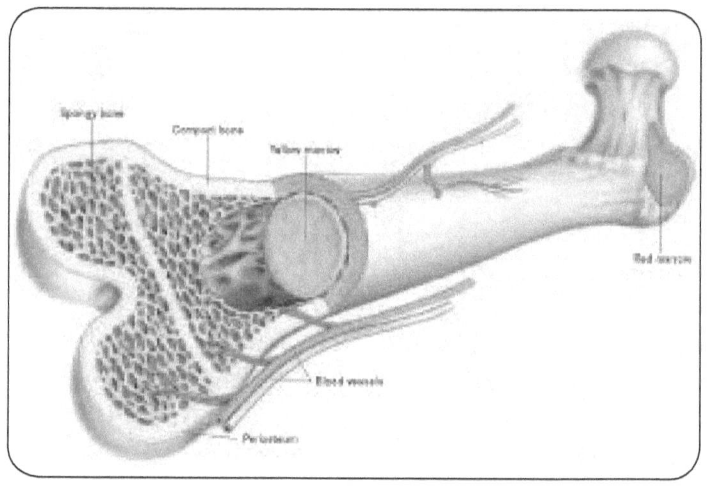

Bone marrow contains two types of stem cells: haemopoietic and stromal cells. Hemopoietic cells produce blood cells, and stromal cells produce fat, cartilage and bone. Bone marrow produces 200 billion new red blood cells every day, along with white blood cells and platelets. During the bone marrow transplant, the cells move back into the bones and start producing blood. They need not be transplanted back into the bone.

❋ ❋ ❋

Spleen: It has multiple roles in the immune system. It filters the blood. Old red blood cells are recycled in the spleen. Platelets and white blood cells are stored. Spleen also helps fight certain kinds of bacteria that cause pneumonia and meningitis. It also creates disease-fighting components of the immune system, including antibodies and lymphocytes.

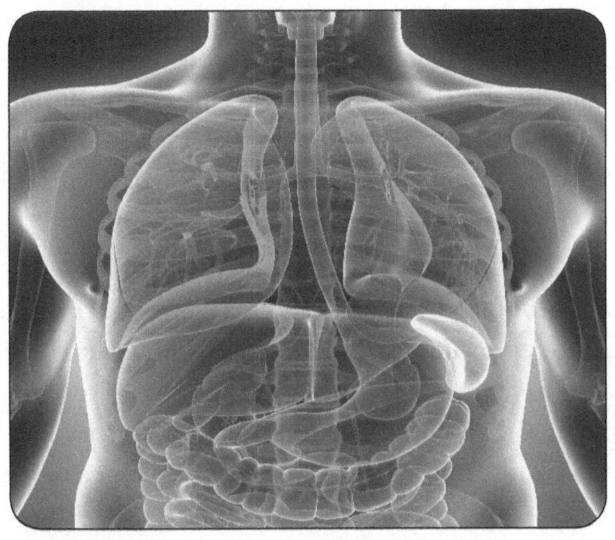

If in case, due to some reason the spleen had to be removed, other organs such as the liver can take over most of the functions. It means we will still be able to cope with most infections. But there's a slight risk that a severe infection may develop quickly.

❁ ❁ ❁

Antibiotics: Antibiotics are drugs that tend to resist bacterial infections. It is a type of antimicrobial agent that is active against bacteria. They do this by killing the bacteria or by preventing them from cloning or reproducing themselves. Any medications that destroy germs in our body are antibiotics. It is the most effective antibacterial agent commonly used to treat and prevent bacterial infections. Antibiotics combat bacterial contamination by destroying their cell walls or covering around bacteria that interfere with bacterial replication.

They can either kill bacteria or slow down their growth. They do this by detecting antigens on the surface of the microbe or the chemicals they produce. The antibodies then mark the degradation of these antigens. There are several cells, proteins and chemicals involved in this attack.

* * *

White blood cells: White blood cells are also referred to as leukocytes (such as B-cells, T-cells and natural killer cells). They protect the body and continue to circulate through the bloodstream to defend against viruses, bacteria and other alien agents that endanger our well-being. They're at war all the time. They initiate an immunity attack when they encounter them. Most of the tests are performed using white blood cells. Since they are so common in our bodies, it is easier to test them for infections. Our body creates various kinds of white blood cells to shield our bodies from different types of invaders. We're going to dig through this principle later. They initiate an immunity attack when they encounter them and the white blood cells are flooded into our bodies. Increased production of white blood cells typically suggests that they are fighting disease.

* * *

The complement system: The complement system, also known as complement cascade, is a part of the immune system that enhances (complements) the ability of antibodies and phagocytic cells to clear microbes and damaged cells from an organism, promote inflammation and attack the pathogen's cell membrane. Typically, it acts as a part of the innate immune system, but it can work with the adaptive immune system if necessary. It consists of several small proteins synthesized by the liver and circulated in the blood. Over 30 proteins and protein fragments make up the complement system, including serum proteins and cell membrane receptors. They account for about 10 per cent of the globulin fraction of the blood serum.

The lymphatic system: The lymphatic system is a network of tissues and organs that eliminates contaminants, waste and other unnecessary materials. It is also known as the Lymphoid gland and is found in all vertebrates as part of the circulatory system and the immune system. Its primary function is to transport lymph, a fluid that comprises white blood cells that fight infection in the body. Primary lymphoid organs manufacture lymphocytes from immature progenitor cells. Thymus and bone marrow are the main lymphoid organs participating in the development and early clonal selection of lymphocyte tissues. Primary lymphoid glands include lymph nodes and spleen. Cancer of the lymphatic system may be primary or secondary. Lymphoma refers to cancer that is caused by lymphatic tissue. Lymphoid leukaemia and lymphoma are also believed to be cancers of the same type of cell lineage.

We know how our immune system behaves. The question is, how do they know that a foreign body has entered and is causing an infection that can cause disease? How does our body discriminate between various cells in our bodies?

For our immune system, a foreign body will be like finding a needle in a haystack. When scientists understood how our immune system works, they also understood the disease from AIDS to auto-immune disorders. Some of the immune system's responses happen quickly, and the infecting agent is contained. Some responses are slower and tailor-made for specific infecting agents.

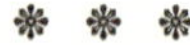

Non-specific immunity: Non-specific immune cells consist of a macrophage, neutrophil or dendritic cell that responds to several antigens. Non-specific immune cells function as the first line of defence against infection or disease. They are still present at the site of infection to fight bacteria or some other infection. They are often referred to as the innate immune response. Macrophages, neutrophils and dendritic cells are all cells of the standard immune system that use phagocytosis and are loaded with Toll-Like Receptors (TLRs). Toll-like receptors are found in cells that recognize different microbial products resulting in more complex immune responses. When a phagocytic cell engulfs bacteria, a phagosome is formed around it, and the whole complex is eventually degraded to the lysosome. Lysosomes have digestive enzymes. They break down excess or worn-out sections of the cells. In this case, there are bacteria and other pathogens. These cells, which participate in non-specific immune system response, cannot differentiate between types of microorganisms but do have the ability to discern between what is self and what is non-self.

❋ ❋ ❋

Specific immunity: Specific immunity, also known as adaptive immunity, is the special immunity for particular pathogens. They are often referred to as the acquired immune system. They have two distinct types of cells (lymphocytes): B cells and T cells. B cells are stimulated to secrete antibodies in the antibody response. These antibodies are receptors, also known as immunoglobulins. They pass through the bloodstream and bind to a foreign antigen, resulting in the antigen to inactivate and hence, hindering the antigen to bind to the host Helper T-cells. Cytotoxic T-cells and B-cells are subject to specific immunity. They work hand-in-hand with non-specific immunity, including macrophages. They tell the T-cells and B-cells that there is an intruder. Acquired immunity is acquired over the body's lifespan and is also called adaptive responses because they prepare the body for a potential reaction. This mechanism is extremely adaptable due to somatic hypermutation. This mechanism allows a small number of genes to generate many different antigen receptors, which are then uniquely expressed on each lymphocyte. Since the gene rearrangement leads to an irreversible change in each cell's DNA, all offspring of that cell inherit genes that encode the same receptor specificity, including the memory B-cells and memory T-cells which are the keys to long-lived specific immunity.

❋ ❋ ❋

Acquired immunity: Acquired immunity is activated in invertebrates when the pathogen escapes the innate immune system and generates a threshold amount of antigen that produces "strong" or "danger" signals that stimulate dendritic cells. Its primary function involves identifying non-self and self-antigens, producing a custom made antigen and developing a memory with which the pathogen can be recognized by memory B-cells and memory T-cells. Think of it as our immune system is made up of three major groups of cells. They're soldier cells, intelligence cells and arms factories. When our simple immune system cannot kill the invaders, the intelligence cells recognize and analyze the threat. The weapon cells then make antibodies to kill cells tailored for a specific kind of infection. It could also take days to evaluate the danger and produce a perfect antibody that may place the patient's life at risk. So, our body remembers the antibody that was used to destroy the antigen. Our body makes memory cells to remember them, which are activated whenever necessary. The question arises, will we ever be immune to everything?

Antibodies have receptors that are used to detect different threats. Our body even has immunity against germs that our body has never seen. How does our body make our cells immune from the germs that our body has never encountered? The distinctive form of the antibody is made up of random shuffling of the genes. The plan is to create enough variations for an antigen to be present to destroy the germ. They can produce new sets of antibodies by using only three unique sets of genetic instructions. It's like a deck of cards; only by choosing a gene from each deck can they make up to 10,000 sets of antibodies. A unique array of DNA letters are inserted between genes that make up 10 million more sets of antigens. If created to adapt, they begin to mutate and tweak their form to keep ahead of the germs. After completing the sets, inserting genes and then mutating themselves, our body can make up to a quintillion (1 and 18 zeros) possible antibodies i.e. 5 million-trillion possible antibody shapes. That's 10 million times the stars in our galaxy. So, could we be immune to anything? Theoretically, yes. But practically, our body is not big enough to hold that many antibodies.

Acquired immunity may also offer long-term security. An individual who has recovered from Measles is protected from measles for their lifetime. In other cases, it does not have a life-long defence, such as chickenpox. The acquired device reaction kills infectious pathogens and any harmful compounds they create. Often acquired immunity cannot differentiate dangerous molecules from harmless foreign molecules. When it cannot discriminate, it affects the body, causing hay fever, asthma or other allergies. Sometimes, the immune system fights and destroys the cells; it's called autoimmune disorders.

Our body is still unable to treat some diseases with such a diverse immune system, or it can take a long time to treat the illness. In some cases, we have medications to help us deal with the disease, allowing us to heal quicker. So, how are these drugs going to work? How are they expected to know where to go and what's the problem?

Medicines are chemicals or compounds used to cure, halt, prevent disease, ease symptoms or help diagnose illnesses. Advances in medications have enabled doctors to cure many diseases and save lives. Every medicine has a specific function, and they change as the disease changes or the advancement of the disease changes. There is always some kind of risk involved in medicine. No matter how safe the treatment is, it can have some side-effects. Side-effects depend on food, alcohol or any other medication. Drugs are prescribed concerning the medical test.

When we swallow a pill, it travels through the stomach and intestine, which disintegrates upon reaching the liver, and then released into the bloodstream. Once released into the bloodstream, it can ride through the whole body. Luckily, our body has a system that is smart enough to get medicines exactly where they're needed. They work like a lock-and-key pattern. Specific medications can be attached to a particular receptor. Our body acts as a lock, and medicines act as a key. As they hit a ride through the blood throughout the body, they keep searching for a lock. They keep searching until they have found it. Each drug is designed to target specific protein molecules called receptors. In pain medications like ibuprofen and acetaminophen, they search out specific receptors generated by pain and inflammation as they course through the bloodstream.

Drug molecules can also bind to an area other than the target, primarily if they are closely related. It can be noticed in cancer treatment by chemotherapy. That's how they detect cancer cells, but they also detect hair cells, which is why many chemotherapy patients lose their hair.

Hair cells also replicate almost as quickly as cancer cells. They lose most of their immunity because it can harm the cells that produce blood like bone marrow.

Drugs administered locally, such as creams for infections or discomfort, have relatively fewer side effects relative to medications that travel through the bloodstream. That is why infants fall sick more often than the elderly, so they are given vaccines to shield them from germs. So, what's a vaccine? What's the difference between the vaccine and the medicine?

Vaccines are distinct from drugs. A significant distinction is that vaccines are delivered before infection, and medications are delivered following an illness. The vaccine can be labelled "what doesn't kill you makes you healthier." In most situations, the vaccine involves an inactivated pathogen that can have a long-lasting effect on our bodies. It is used to prepare the immune system so that when the real pathogen of the same form threatens to attack our bodies, our bodies will be able to protect itself against major damage or minor damage. Different vaccines have different lifespans. Vaccines provided for Measles can last a lifetime in more than 96 per cent of vaccines. Vaccines given for mumps can last over ten years in 90 per cent of vaccines. Most vaccines stay longer than 90 per cent and are protected for more than 15-20 years. This is one of the reasons that vaccines are given periodically in all vertebrates.

Vaccines are used in a variety of ways. Travellers preparing to visit places where such diseases are prevalent, such as typhoid fever or yellow fever, are given brief warnings shortly before the ride. Vaccines such as influenza vaccines or flu vaccinations are usually offered to particular classes of individuals, such as older adults and those at high risk of contracting or complicating influenza. Rabies vaccine is administered when we are known to be exposed to the virus that causes the infection like a dog bite. Certain vaccines are given to almost everyone, such as preventing diphtheria, tetanus, polio and measles.

Children routinely get a set of vaccines that begin at birth. These vaccines defend against hepatitis B, diphtheria, tetanus, whooping cough, measles, mumps, German measles, chickenpox, polio, pneumococcal, Haemophilus influenza type b (Hib) and hepatitis A. According to a particular timetable, the American Academy advises this sequence of vaccines of Family Physicists, the American Academy of Paediatrics, and Centers for Disease Control and Prevention. It is required in all states before schooling. All states have an exemption for people who have medical disorders, such as cancer patients. However, in some states, there is an exception to regional beliefs.

It is a religious practice that infants need not be vaccinated. If you want to save a few bucks and risk your children being sick, then you might leave your child unvaccinated. Vaccines have side-effects. It is estimated that 0.0001 per cent of infants, which is 1 in 10,000, have life-threatening experience with the vaccine due to allergies from vaccines. However, the positives outweigh the side-effects. Suppose babies are not given the primary vaccine. In that case, the risk factor is expected to rise from about 5 per cent to 20 per cent for measles; it is comparatively greater than 0.0001 per cent. 95 per cent of people must be vaccinated to have herd immunity for measles. Suppose the infant is resistant to the vaccine and is not vaccinated. In that case, it might not be a matter of concern, but if everybody thinks the same and the percentages fall below 95 per cent, the chance of infection increases, and it then becomes a matter of concern. This is not only the case with measles but also the same with all the vaccinations.

In infants, mothers feed milk for about one year so that the antibiotics from their mothers' milk are absorbed by the baby's body and can be used to combat pathogens. If a pathogen has never infected the mother, she will not have an antibody and will not pass on the pathogen. That's why infants are vaccinated after birth.

There is another method in which immunity is passed from one human to another is called plasma transfusion. Our immune cells are present in the plasma that runs through the blood. Plasma is extracted from individuals with antibodies, and under laboratory conditions, the antibodies are nurtured and replicated. Then the antibody is injected into the person who was infected. The sick person's body takes and replicates the antibody and tries to combat the infection. We have accomplished this in real life. When the Spanish flu occurred in 1918, about 500 million people died. The survivors were immune to the virus. When the Spanish flu returned in 2009, 1918 survivors' antibodies were used to keep other individuals healthy. But the germs keep mutating, and our immune system still needs to adapt. That's why we have to take a flu virus short every year.

Having such evolved immune systems, why do we have a pandemic? To understand why we need to understand what a pandemic is? Let me take you to my next chapter, "Pandemic."

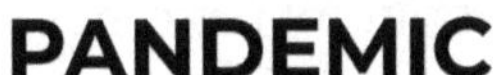
PANDEMIC

It is one of the words everyone can relate to nowadays. About a year ago, no one in this world would have thought that the darkest nightmare might come true. Well, it is not for me, since I am having fun sitting home, working from home, working out and occasionally going out for a breather. I have everything I want. I get paid to work from home, and I eat nutritious food. I have stopped eating outside food for about seven months, and I have lost about 6 pounds working out from home. Well, not everyone has the same story. A survey was conducted where 2000 people were asked to fill out a study, and the data revealed that about 59 per cent of people are happily working from home and 41 per cent of the people are eager to continue working from home. Well, I am one of them. The problem starts when the actual numbers come up.

Approximately, only 10 per cent of the people are working from home in India. In the U.S., only seven per cent of the people were working from home until 2017. 64 per cent of U.S. employees work from home now, while U.S. data include only office workers. 59 per cent of U.S. workers who have worked from home during the coronavirus pandemic would prefer to continue to work remotely as much as possible once public health restrictions are lifted. In contrast, 41 per cent would choose to return to their workplace or office to work, as they did before the crisis. This number remains the same in most countries. But the percentage of people working from home varies from country to country.

Every region is subject to substantial growth downgrades. East Asia and the Pacific will grow by a scant 0.5 per cent. South Asia will contract by 2.7 per cent, Sub-Saharan Africa by 2.8 per cent, Middle East and North Africa by 4.2 per cent, Europe and Central Asia by 4.7 per cent, and Latin America by 7.2 per cent. These downturns are expected to reverse years of progress towards development goals and trip tens of millions of people back into extreme poverty; on average, the world's GDP dropped by 4.5 per cent.

The consequences of the pandemic can be seen for a long time. Many countries took decades to grow their economic GDP, and it was crushed in six months. Having such an impact on the roots, the question arises, what is a pandemic? When was it declared that it is a pandemic? Why does it have so many effects? Well, to understand those, we must understand what a pandemic is.

The pandemic is defined as "an epidemic occurring worldwide, or over an extensive area, crossing international boundaries and usually affecting many people." It can happen due to viruses, bacteria or any other harmful agent. By this definition, pandemics can occur annually in each of the temperate southern and northern hemispheres. These seasonal epidemics cross international boundaries and affect a large number of people. However, seasonal epidemics are not considered pandemics. Seasonal pandemics can also cause viral, including fever, during the rainy season or any other season. These pandemics mostly occur in moderate temperatures where a bacterium or a virus can thrive easily. A pandemic is a near-global disease outbreak when multiple countries are infected.

The major difference between seasonal-pandemic and pandemic is, in most cases, there are medicines available for a seasonal pandemic. Even if there are no available medicines, the seasonal pandemic will pass away with the season and might return the following year. It is not the same case with the pandemic because, in most cases, there are no available medicines and it does not pass away just as easily. In most cases, it comes when a virus or a bacterium jumps from species to species. A pandemic can be easily confused with an epidemic, endemic or outbreak.

"A widespread occurrence of an infectious disease in a community at a particular time" is called an epidemic. For example, in meningococcal infections, an attack rate over 15 cases per 1,00,000 people for two consecutive weeks is considered an epidemic. An epidemic can be confined to a location; however, if it spreads to other countries or continents and affects a substantial number of people, then it can be termed as a pandemic.

"A disease or condition regularly found among particular people or in a certain area" is called an endemic. In the UK, chickenpox is considered endemic, but malaria is not. While in Africa, it is most common to say AIDS as an endemic. It is the use of the word in its etymological rather than an epidemiological form. AIDS cases are increasing, so the disease is not in a steady endemic state. The spread of AIDS in Africa can be correctly called an epidemic. In this state neither the infection dies nor does the population of the infected people increase exponentially. They're just balanced that neither the viruses die nor they are too successful.

A sudden increase in occurrences of a disease at a particular time and place is called an outbreak. It may affect small and localized groups or impact thousands of people across the country. Outbreaks include epidemics, which are normally only used for infectious diseases and diseases with an environmental origin, such as water or food-borne disease. They may affect a group of countries or a region. The terms "outbreak" and "epidemic" have often been interchanged.

Being so dangerous, is COVID the first pandemic outbreak we had? If not, what are they? Starting from 430 BC (Antonine Plague) to 2020 (Corona Virus) to date, we have had many notable and nonnotable outbreaks. Let's go through a couple of them.

The Plague of Athens: It was an epidemic that devastated Athens' city-state in ancient Greece during the second year of the Peloponnesian War. The plague killed an estimated 75,000 to 100,000 people. It is believed to have entered Athens through Piraeus, the city's port and sole source of food and supplies. Symptoms included fever, thirst, bloody throat and tongue, red skin and lesions. The disease, suspected to have been typhoid fever, weakened the Athenians significantly and was a significant factor in their Spartans' defeat. The plague returned twice in 429 BC and in the winter of 427/426 BC. Some 30 pathogens were suspected of having caused the plague. One of the reasons why this outbreak was fatal is the sheer contagiousness of the illness. Those who tended to the illness were most vulnerable to catching the disease.

Many people were left to die alone because no one was willing to take the risk of caring for them. The dead were piled on top of each other, left to rot or shoved into mass graves. Sometimes, the dead had to be burnt in heaps, and a new body was dumped on it. The lucky-enough survivors had developed immunity and would later become caretakers for those who fell ill. Mass graves of about 1,000 tombs were built, dated between 430 and 426 BC. The plague caused the largest recorded loss of life in ancient Greece.

Antonine Plague: The epidemic from 165 to 180 AD, also known as the Epidemic of Galen (after Galen, the doctor who named the Plague), was an ancient pandemic introduced to the Roman Empire by soldiers returning from the Near East campaigns. Symptoms included fever, sore throat, diarrhoea and if the patient lived long enough, then pus-filled sores. Scholars also believed that it could be smallpox or measles. The Roman emperor, Lucius Verus, also died in 169 AD due to this plague. Approximately 5 million civilians died, which was one-third of the population in some places, and ravaged the Roman army. Australian sinologist and historian Rafe de Crespigny suggests that the plague may have also occurred in Eastern Han China before 166 AD due to accounts of plague in Chinese documents.

The Plague of Cyprian: This pandemic influenced the Roman Empire from 249 to 262 AD. It is considered to be the same as the Antonine Plague. It was like a second plague. This plague has seriously damaged the Roman army, triggering food problems and workforce shortages. Symptoms of the plague included diarrhoea, vomiting, ulcers in the stomach, fever and gangrenous hands and legs. Pests contain smallpox, pandemic influenza, and infectious haemorrhagic fever (filoviruses) such as the Ebola virus. About 5,000 people were sick a day at the height of the epidemic and were said to have died in Rome. According to Kyle Harper, a historian, the epidemic had almost stopped in the Roman Empire.

The Plague of Justinian: This pandemic struck during the sixth century and is estimated to have killed about 30 to 50 million people, which was about half of the world's population at the time as it spread across Asia, North Africa, Arabia and Europe. Some theories suggest this plague was similar to that of the Black Death that struck between 1347 and 1351, some 800 years later, killing 50 million Europeans alone. Both plagues were spread to humans by rodents whose fleas carried the bacteria. This pandemic is also considered the beginning of the first plague pandemic. This contagious disease is caused by the bacterium called Yersinia pestis.

The plague of Justinian is meant to kill about a fifth of the population of the imperial capital and to be named after the Roman emperor in Constantinople. The Byzantine historian Procopius first reported the epidemic in 541 from the port of Pelusium, near Suez in Egypt. According to contemporary sources, the outbreak in Constantinople was thought to have been carried to the city by infected rats on grain ships arriving from Egypt. Genetic studies of the modern and ancient Yersinia pestis DNA suggest that it originated from Central Asia. The root-level existing strains of the bacterium as a whole species are found in Qinghai, China.

Black Death: This was the deadliest epidemic known to humanity. It was known to exist after 800 years of the Plague of Justinian. It happened from 1347 to 1351. It was the beginning of the second plague pandemic. The epidemic created religious, social and economic disturbances, with intense effects on European history. It most likely originated in Central Asia or East Asia, from where it travelled along the Silk Road, reaching Crimea by 1347. From there, it travelled on fleas, rats and other rodents on merchant ships spreading throughout the Mediterranean Basin and reaching Africa, Western Asia and the rest of Europe via Constantinople, Sicily and the Italian Peninsula. It is estimated to have killed 30 per cent to 60 per cent of Europe's population. In total, the plague reduced the world population to about 475 million to 350–375 million in the 14th century. The outbreaks of the plague recurred in various parts around the world until the early 19th century. This plague is the first to infect humans in Europe and Asia in the late Neolithic and early Bronze Age.

In 2018, researchers found evidence of Yersinia pestis in an ancient Swedish tomb, which is associated with the "Neolithic decline" around 3000 BCE, in which European populations fell significantly. Due to climatic changes in Asia, rodents began to flee the dried-out grasslands to the most populated areas, spreading the disease. Philip VI of France blamed the heavens in conjunction with three planets that had caused "great pestilence in the air" (caused due to bad air or black air).

Third plague pandemic: This pandemic was a significant plague pandemic caused due to fleas that began in Yunnan, China, in 1855 during the fifth year of the Xianfeng Emperor of the Qing Dynasty. Symptoms include swollen lymph nodes, which can be as large as chicken eggs, in the groin, armpit or neck. It led to the deaths of more than 12 million people in India and China, with about 10 million killed in India alone. The pandemic is considered to be active until 1960 when the worldwide casualties dropped to 200 per year.

The natural reservoir for plague is in western Yunnan and is still an ongoing health risk. The global distribution chart shows that the plague started from Beihai, Qing China, in 1882 to the Russian Empire/ Soviet Union in 1900–1927. The last significant outbreak of plague associated with the pandemic occurred in Peru and Argentina in 1945. This pandemic is also meant to be caused due to Yersinia pestis, just like the Black Death and the Plague of Justinian. That's why this is known as the third plague. French bacteriologist Alexandre Yersin isolated the bacterium by using insecticides and the use of antibiotics, which eventually led to plague vaccines. In 1898, French researcher Paul-Louis Simond demonstrated the role of fleas as vectors. Today, rare cases of plague still occur in the western United States.

1918 flu pandemic: 1918 flu is also known as the Spanish flu virus or the H1N1 influenza A virus. It lasted from February 1918 until April 1920. Around 500 million people were infected, almost a third of the world's population, and the total death rate was between 17 million and 50 million, making it one of the deadliest pandemics in modern history. The first observations of infection and death were recorded in the United States. Many influenza viruses kill the very young and the very old. The percentage of survivors who were young adults was higher. The 2009 swine flu pandemic was followed by the Spanish flu.

Both pandemics were caused due to the same type of virus. Spain was not involved in the war and therefore had not imposed wartime censorship. Newspapers were free to report the epidemic's effects. There were widely spread stories which created a false impression that Spain was severely hit. Different places named it differently. In Senegal, it was called 'the Brazilian flu' and in Brazil, 'the German flu.' At the same time, in Poland, it is known as 'the Bolshevik disease.' 4 March 1918 is marked as the start of the pandemic with a recording of the case of Albert Gitchell, an army cook at Camp Funston in Kansas, U.S., despite there likely having been cases before him. As the U.S. entered World War One, the disease quickly spread like wildfire.

Asian flu: This was the 1956-1958 influenza pandemic caused due to Influenza A virus subtype H2N2. It was a combination of Avian Influenza (probably from a duck) and the human influenza virus. The first case was reported in Guizhou, a landlocked province in the southwest of the People's Republic of China, in early 1956 or early 1957. The neighbouring area of Yunnan reported that they were affected before the end of February. On 17 April, The Times reported that "an influenza epidemic has affected thousands of Hong Kong residents." In Taiwan, 100,000 were affected by mid-May, and India suffered a million cases by June. In late June, the pandemic reached the United Kingdom. It reached the United States by the end of June 1957. The first wave proved fatal among children who had just started school after the summer break, whereas the second wave, which came during January and February of 1958, proved fatal among elderly people.

The Public Health Service released the virus culture to vaccine manufacturers on 12 May 1957. The vaccine entered trials at Fort Ord on July 26 and Lowry Air Force Base on July 29. The number of deaths in England and Wales was estimated to be 600 deaths per week by the end of 17 October. H2N2 influenza virus continued to be transmitted until 1968 when it transformed into influenza A virus subtype H3N2, the cause of the 1968 influenza pandemic.

HIV/AIDS: It is also known as human immunodeficiency virus infection and acquired immune deficiency syndrome. This virus is expected to attack our immune system. When we have a disease or an outer body attacking our body, our immune system attacks it and protects us from the threats. Human immunodeficiency viruses are two species of Lentivirus, which overtime mutated to form HIV. There may not be any prolonged symptoms of the influenza-like illness for at least a brief period of time.

As the virus keeps interfering more with the immune system, it increases the risk of developing common infections, whereas it will be difficult to grow the infection in other people. These late symptoms of the disease are referred to as acquired immunodeficiency syndrome (AIDS), which leads to unintended weight loss. They are spread primarily by unprotected sex, contaminated blood transfusions, hypodermic needles and from mother to child during pregnancy, delivery or breastfeeding. HIV is a member of a group of viruses known as retroviruses. That is why some bodily fluids, such as saliva, sweat and tears, do not transmit the virus. The first known case of human infection with HIV-1 was identified in a blood sample obtained in 1959 from a man in Kinshasa, the Democratic Republic of the Congo. Scientists have established the species of chimpanzee in West Africa as a vector of HIV infection in humans. They claim that the chimpanzee form of the immunodeficiency virus (called the Simian Immunodeficiency Virus or SIV) was most likely transferred to humans and transformed into HIV after humans killed these chimpanzees for meat and came into touch with their contaminated blood.

Over the decades, the virus slowly spread across Africa and later into other parts of the world. Genetic analysis of this blood sample suggested that HIV-1 may have stemmed from a single virus in the late 1940s or early 1950s. In 2018, about 37.9 million people were living with HIV, and it resulted in 7,70,000 deaths. An estimated 20.6 million of these live in eastern and southern Africa. Between the times AIDS was identified (in early 1980s) and 2018, the disease caused an estimated 32 million deaths worldwide, which is why AIDS is considered a pandemic. The disease has become subject to many controversies involving religion, including the Catholic Church's position not to support condom use as prevention. There are three main stages of HIV infection: acute infection, clinical latency and AIDS.

SARS: It is also known as the severe acute respiratory syndrome or SARS-CoV-1. It is a respiratory disease that originated from pathogens that jump from animals to humans. In late 2017, Chinese scientists traced the virus through the intermediary of Asian palm civets to cave-dwelling horseshoe bats in Yunnan. It was a relatively rare disease. However, the case fatality rate was 11 per cent, with worldwide reported cases being 8,422. The primary route of transmission is the contact of the mucous membranes with respiratory droplets or fomites. While diarrhoea is common in people with SARS, the fecal-oral course does not appear to be a common transmission mode. As SARS infects the lungs and is a virus, it cannot be killed using antibiotics. The treatment is mainly supportive with antipyretics, supplemental oxygen and mechanical ventilation. At the same time, Ribavirin is commonly used to treat SARS. As of 2020, there is no effective vaccine or cure for SARS, which is both effective and safe for humans. A farmer from Shunde, Foshan, Guangdong, was treated and was the first-known patient in the First People's Hospital of Foshan. The patient died soon after, and no definite diagnosis was made on the cause of death.

Despite actions to control the pandemic, Chinese government officials did not inform the WHO about the break until February 2003. This lack of openness caused the delay in controlling the pandemic, resulting in the criticism of the People's Republic of China from the international community. China officially apologized for the slowness in dealing with the pandemic. An American businessman, Johnny Chen, travelling from China to Singapore, was affected with pneumonia-like symptoms. The plane stopped in Hanoi, Vietnam, where the victim died in Hanoi French Hospital. The doctors who treated the patient were noticed to have the same symptoms. Later the Italian doctor Carlo Urbani identified the threat and communicated it to the WHO and the Vietnamese government. Global health professionals saw SARS as a wake-up call to improve outbreak responses, and lessons from the pandemic were used to keep diseases like H1N1, Ebola and Zika under control.

COVID-19: It is also known as the severe acute respiratory syndrome coronavirus or SARS-CoV-2. Severe acute respiratory syndrome coronavirus 2 (SARS-CoV-2) is a novel severe acute respiratory syndrome coronavirus, which is why it is called a novel coronavirus. It is a respiratory disease that originated from pathogens that jump from animals to humans. It was first identified in Wuhan, Hubei, China in December 2019 and has been ongoing since then. As of 30 September 2020, more than 33.5 million cases have been reported across 188 countries and territories with more than 1 million deaths; more than 23.2 million people have recovered. Some common symptoms include fever, cough, fatigue, shortness of breath or breathing difficulties, and loss of smell and taste. Symptoms may vary slightly from person to person. The disease spreads between people as they come in close physical contact. The primary source of transamination is via small droplets or particles such as aerosols, produced after an infected person breathes, coughs, sneezes, talks or sings. That is the reason why masks are requested to be worn at all times when you come in close proximity with others.

People remain infectious in moderate cases for 7–12 days and up to two weeks in severe cases. It can transmit when it is symptomatic, which is about two days before developing symptoms. A July 2020 systematic review found that the proportion of asymptomatic cases ranged from 6 per cent to 41 per cent. Genetic analysis has revealed that coronavirus genetically clusters with the genus Betacoronavirus, in subgenus Sarbecovirus (lineage B), and two bat-derived strains. It is 96 per cent identical to the whole genome of the coronavirus samples obtained from the bat species.

Currently, there are no effective medicines for coronavirus. But there are specific methods prescribed by WHO to control the spread and cure the patients. 2.3 per cent of the affected people passed away. 5 per cent are in critical condition, 14 per cent are in severe condition and 81 per cent are mild cases. The global mortality rate was about 3.0 per cent whereas 11 per cent was in SARS. A higher mortality rate was noticed in China and Italy. The death rate in men was expected to be 2.8 per cent and 1.7 per cent in women. In Europe, 57 per cent of the infected people were men, and 72 per cent of those who died were men.

These were just some of the notable pandemics. The list goes on, including the 11th century: Leprosy, 1492: The Columbian Exchange, 1665: The Great Plague of London, 1817: First Cholera Pandemic, 1875: Fiji Measles Pandemic and 1889: Russian Flu. If we notice, by the 18th century, we've had about eight pandemics, and since the 18th century, we've had nine pandemics. Why do we see such drastic change? Has anything changed? If yes, what has changed?

There are many factors that affect the start, spread and end of pandemics. One of the significant factors that affect the beginning and spread of the pandemic is the world population or the population of a region and the environmental factors. Many factors affect or encourage the start, and many can expedite the process. One of the major driving factors is the environment. All the pathogens come from somewhere.

Most of the pandemics caused are due to pathogens jumping from organism to organism, mainly from animals to humans. When a virus jumps from an animal to a human, it mutates into millions of the virus. Every once in a while, it hits the jackpot and infects the organisms. The virus not only jumps from other animals to humans but also jumps from humans to animals. However, it mostly affects humans. The question stands, why? The answer is we are everywhere. Yes, you heard it right. We interact with all the animals available in the world. Humans can be found in every corner of the world.

When we interact with most of the animals in the world, the possibility of the virus to mutate increases. A cat living in Africa might have a virus that can infect a lion in Asia since they live so far. It is difficult for them to come in contact, but this is not the case with us. Remember, we are everywhere.

The mode of infection mostly depends on the part the virus infects and the rate at which it replicates itself. Most of the viruses that transmit through mostly infect the lungs, and the viruses that infect the immune system are transmitted mainly through blood transfusion or by sex. That is the same reason why the transamination of HIV is higher in females than in men. The bodily fluids can quickly move from the male genitalia to the female genitalia, and it has white blood cells. White blood cells are also not exposed to the open air to transmit the virus through the air. COVID-19 replicates in our lungs, and lungs breathe air. So, the virus moves through the air. Since it moves through the air, it spreads faster and can be contracted faster. Fluid builds up in the lungs can prove fatal since it reduces the amount of air that we can breathe, in turn reducing the amount of oxygen that reaches the body. Since there is no medicine for COVID-19, it is challenging to cure. One of the major reasons is that our body will not get enough time to develop immunity to the virus, leading to death.

One of the significant factors that affects a pandemic is hygiene. Having poor hygiene increases the probability of the start of a deadly pandemic. Not long ago, in the second half of the nineteenth century, hygiene and sanitation were at the forefront of the struggle against illness and disease. Having a clean neighbourhood also means having more fresh air and a healthy environment.

Some of the mental factors that affect a pandemic are distraction, fear, stress, fatigue, rushing and uncertainty.

Fear can lead to erratic or unpredictable decision-making. The fear of contracting a disease may also cause workers to appear standoffish, withdrawn and less willing to step in to help co-workers. Employees may be so focused on avoiding contact with others that they'll be less receptive to the dangers of familiar physical hazards. Fear triggers the flight and fight process, which are survival instincts. In-flight or fight process, we tend to save ourselves in most cases.

The news seems to change by the hour. The media tell us how many people are sick or dead, which states plan on re-opening and in what capacity, and which politician is arguing for a particular policy aimed at curbing the pandemic's societal damage. It's impossible not to be distracted these days. But just because it's an understandable state of affairs, it doesn't mean it's any less risky. Health workers in both sectors should be mindful that the vast majority of their workforce is more overwhelmed than normal.

Although this may not be the most obvious problem, persistent stress will drastically affect the way people behave in the workplace. It influences how employees handle information and make safety choices. It also affects routine activities and routines such as wearing PPE masks, gloves or other protective clothing. Stress can be difficult to detect because it may always be unseen, or otherwise; the signs can seem to suggest other human causes, such as irritation, exhaustion or sickness. So, that makes depression all the more difficult to address. All told, tension is one of the most serious safety issues caused by the pandemic.

Fatigue is one of the reasons that human causes are so stealthy that they are amplified in many forms. Not only can their consequences layer on top of each other, but it's riskier to be interrupted and hurried than to be distracted and work at an average pace. Moreover, one human aspect can also be a catalyst that can cause more to happen. This is particularly true when it comes to exhaustion. A typical symptom of anxiety, tension and general confusion about the future is the challenge of sleeping, resulting in exhaustion. It brings millions of people to work in states of tension, exhaustion and anxiety. If you're counting, then that's three separate risk-elevating states of mind that impact workers before they strike for their shift. There may also be other causes of exhaustion, especially in sectors that have increased demand to accommodate an increase in orders or in places of work that have decreased the number of workers on the floor due to lay-offs or social distance steps. In cases like these, people may need to work harder or longer than usual, which can lead to fatigue.

Change in the workplace can not only cause fatigue in particular but, cause the workers to work at a faster pace to meet the global product demand at a lower wage. There are other reasons for rushing. Since their jobs are inline, which can increase their probability of getting fired, they tend to work harder. Rushing at the workplace can reduce the quality of the product. Rushing over the work can also cause general stress.

Eventually, every company needs to start working. When the workers return to the workplace, not everything will be the same. To go with the regulation of the pandemic, there will be sanitization and social distancing. This change in the work environment is uncertain; some of the sudden changes might lead to anxiety. Uncertainty is an often overlooked but potentially dangerous state of mind. Workers are not aware of what they must do when their co-workers go down. This uncertainty in workers can lead to panic among the workers as they do not know where they will get the answers.

One of the significant factors that affects the beginning of a pandemic is the control and the pandemic in the initial stages. A pandemic is called a pandemic when it crosses the country border and affects many people. Controlling the pandemic in the initial stage can be termed as an epidemic. To manage a pandemic in the initial stage, it is necessary to identify the pandemic. One of the best methods to identify a pandemic is people's common symptoms in a region of the area.

Most of the infections have typical symptoms. Symptoms might show up at different times, but they are mostly the same. As symptoms of more than 5 per cent match in a respective area and the disease seems to be contagious, the area should be monitored for contaminants, infections or other environmental factors that can cause a group or a community ill. Based on the analysis of the data, if it comes out that it is a pandemic, then it is essential to understand how the disease spreads. Suppose the disease is unable to infect a new host, the spreading stops. As the spreading stops, the pandemic comes to an end. One of the major strategies to fight pandemic is "flattening the curve."

The first objective of a pandemic is to increase appropriate care facilities. Flattening the curve is a strategy based on the same principle. This strategy was used during SARS-CoV-2 and is used in COVID-19 pandemic. The curve is an epidemic curve, a visual representation of the number of infected people needing health care over time. During an epidemic, the health care system can break down when the number of people infected exceeds the healthcare system's ability to take care of them. Flattening the curve means slowing the spread of the pandemic so that the government gets enough time to increase the hospitals' capacity.

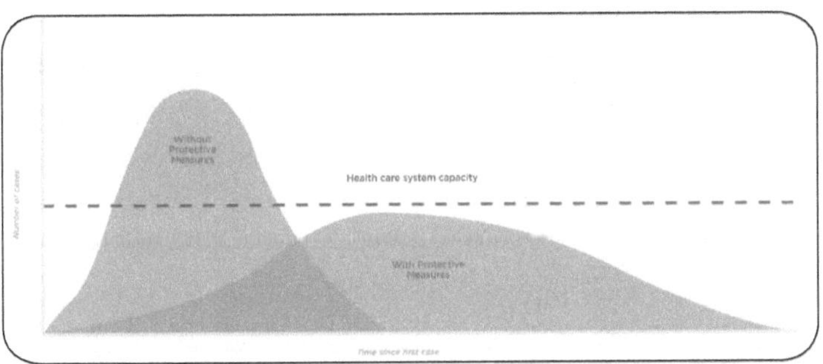

The graph above shows two curves. The orange curve is without preventive action, and the blue curve is with preventative measure. The flatter the blue curve, the health care services can take better care of patients. Flattening the curve depends on mitigation methods, such as following social distancing. 'Flatten the curve' deals with two things: keeping the health care system from getting overrun and slowing down the risk of infection.

So, there aren't too many cases that need hospitalizing. It tends to improve the ability of the hospital system to accommodate a significant number of patients. In the case of the COVID-19 pandemic, the major steps were to expand the number of available ICU beds and ventilators in structural shortages. Non-medical methods such as handwashing, social distancing, separation of the sick, and disinfection are some of the features used to control the virus's spread. The level of strictness of these factors defines the spread of the infection.

Understanding and encouraging people to understand the pandemic is the first step in managing the pandemic. If people are sceptical about the magnitude of the disease and its risks, the virus can spread like wildfire. Without adequate understanding, no appropriate action can be taken by people to control the disease. It can have a negative impact on the country. Live reports on pandemic cases must include the rate of transmission, the mortality rate and the overall number of infections. It is, therefore, essential to exchange information about how to control the spread pandemic.

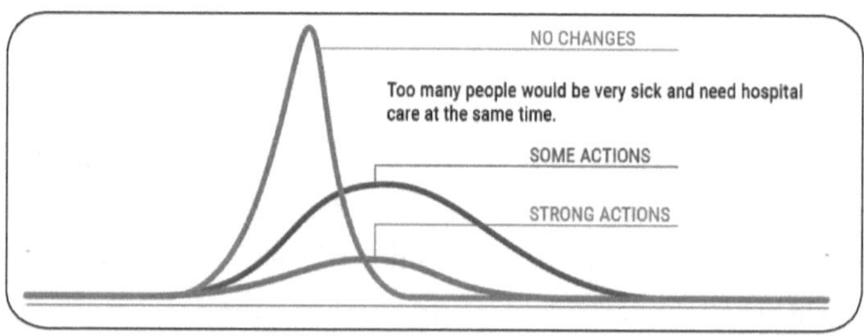

In the above graph, you can see three curves with the variation in the country's strictness. Another factor that affects the spread of the pandemic is knowledge and understanding.

Essential protections, such as masks and gloves, should be a compulsion during the pandemic along with social distancing. Eatables can be purchased in bulk for at least a week. News media must report facts about the pandemic, such as its symptoms, how it progresses and its containment.

The Hindu has reported a piece of news about Mr Shaikh Abdullah, who is 67 years old. Every day, the self-proclaimed activist sets out at 10.30 a.m. on his bicycle from his home on Nathar Shah Mosque Road, which is in Tiruchirappalli, also called Tiruchi or Trichy in Tamil Nadu, which lies in southern parts of India. He visits areas like Central Bus Stand, Railway Junction, Cantonment, Collectorate, Alwarthope and Palakkarai before returning home at 3 p.m.

As published by The Hindu, he quoted, "I want the public to take the government's warnings about COVID-19 seriously. Wherever I go, I find many people sceptical about the magnitude of the disease and dangers posed by it. They keep crowding against the advice given by the authorities. That's why I take these messages to the people and make short speeches. People stop to listen to my short speeches and read the charts I have put up on my cycle. If I had permission, I could ride farther into places like Srirangam and Ariyamangalam. In the evening, I try and cycle into the shopping areas near my home. You have to get the message across even though the weather is so hot."

Everything in this world has a beginning. So, the question arises, where did this pandemic start? To understand the beginning of this pandemic in-depth, let me take you to my next chapter, "Everything Comes From Somewhere."

EVERYTHING COMES FROM SOMEWHERE

Viruses that start the pandemic have to come from somewhere. To know where the beginning of this pandemic is we must understand what it is. So, what is coronavirus? As we discussed earlier, a coronavirus is a group of retroviruses that can infect mammals and birds. Most commonly, they cause respiratory tract infections that can range from mild to lethal. In most mild cases in humans, it causes the common cold, and in most fatal cases, it includes fever, cough, fatigue, shortness of breath, and loss of smell and taste. Lethal viruses include SARS, MERS, and COVID-19.

In animals like cows and pigs, they cause diarrhoea, while in mice, they cause hepatitis and encephalomyelitis. There are as yet no vaccines or antiviral drugs to prevent or treat human coronavirus infections. It enveloped a positive-sense single-stranded RNA genome with a nucleocapsid (capsid of a virus with the enclosed nucleic acid) of helical symmetry.

The genome size of coronaviruses ranges from approximately 26 to 32 kilobases, one of the largest among RNA viruses. The name "coronavirus" is derived from the Latin corona, meaning "crown" or "wreath," which is itself borrowed from the Greek word "garland or wreath." The most recent common ancestor of all coronavirus is estimated to be as recent as 8000 BC, although some theories suggest that it existed around 55 million years ago or possibly more. Bats and birds are the ultimate reservoirs as they are warm-blooded vertebrates.

Alphacoronaviruses and betacoronaviruses live in Bats, and Gammacoronaviruses and deltacoronaviruses live in birds. Most coronavirus that had infected humans shared a common ancestor with bats. But the question stands, why don't bats get infected? The answer lies in the environment they live in and their ability to fly. Bats often live in an environment that helps a virus to grow. Often exposed to harmful and deadly pathogens, they have a strong immune system and are at a never-ending war with pathogens and the virus. Another reason why a bat can survive is its ability to fly. When bats fly, their body temperature can reach up to 37.77°C to 40.55°C or 100°F to 105°F. In most mammals, it's the temperature that causes fever. At 37.00 degrees Celsius the virus can survive for up to 2 days. At 56.00 degrees Centigrade, the virus can survive up to 15 min. Many viruses that reach a temperature of 37°C can die in a short time also. During the flight, bats increase their metabolic rate from 15 times to 16 times higher than non-flying bats.

When the bat starts flying, the body temperature rises exponentially. The temperature increases suddenly; thus, it has a higher chance of killing the virus on the flight or causing some severe damage, which can then be killed by their body's immune system. Researchers hope that their study will help the scientific community analyze the bats' immuno-response and find ways to develop therapies that could help humans fight against such diseases in the future. This combination keeps the virus sustaining and in check. This virus is found in bats and animals.

The first cases of coronavirus in animals occurred in 1920, which caused acute respiratory infection of domesticated chickens in North America. Arthur Schalk and M.C. Hawn provided the first detailed study documenting a recent respiratory epidemic in chickens in North Dakota in 1931. The strain is known as the Contagious Bronchitis Strain (IBV). It was first grown in the laboratories in 1937. At the end of the 1940s, two other animal coronaviruses, JHM, affected by brain inflammation (murine encephalitis), and the hepatitis-induced mouse hepatitis virus (MHV), were detected in mice. Back then, researchers did not know that the three viruses were linked to each other. Human coronaviruses were discovered in the 1960s. The mortality rate for this infection in newborn babies was about 40-90 per cent.

Coronaviruses are large, roughly spherical particles with unique surface projections like thorns. They vary in size to an average length of 125 nm, with sizes ranging from 50 to 200 nm. The viral envelope is made up of a thin polar membrane made of two layers of lipid molecules. It mainly consists of three types of protein. They include S, also called structural protein, which interacts with the host protein, M, called membrane protein, and E, also called an envelope. Together M and E proteins are called structural proteins as they form the structure of the virus.

Spikes are the most distinguishing feature of coronaviruses. They consist of S protein, which has 270 to 510 amino acids. Each spike is about 20 nm and used for receptor-binding and membrane fusion between the virus and host cell. They have S protein; the S protein is, in turn, composed of S1 and S2 protein. S1 forms a spike that binds the receptors, and S2 includes the stem that anchors the spike in the viral envelope, enabling fusion, which helps the virus enter the cell. S1 protein is the most critical component in terms of infection as they are responsible for identifying the binding receptors. They possess two major domains named the N-terminal domain (S1-NTD) and the C-terminal domain (S1-CTD). They both serve as receptor binding domains. NDT recognizes the binding sugars in the host cells' surface, and CTD's are responsible for the protein receptors.

M protein is the structural protein of the envelope and provides its oval shape. It has 218 to 263 amino acid residues. It forms a layer of 7.8 nm thickness with three domains, such as a short N-terminal ectodomain, a triple-spanning transmembrane domain and a C-terminal endodomain. The C-terminal part forms a matrix-like lattice that adds to the extra-thickness of the envelope. M protein is crucial in the virus's life cycle, such as during assembly, budding, envelope formation and pathogenesis.

E proteins are minor structural proteins and vary highly from species to species. There are only about 20 E proteins in coronavirus. They have 76 to 109 amino acids. They have a particular functional region for securing their position within the cellular membrane and have two domains: the transmembrane domain and the extramembrane C-terminal domain. They are responsible for virion assembly, morphogenesis (budding) and intracellular trafficking.

The replication begins when the infection starts, and it starts when the spike protein attaches to the protein receptor. After the attachment, a protein from the host called protease gets activated, which breaks down the protein into smaller chunks of the amino acids. Host protease availability and activation availability allows the virus to enter through endocytosis or direct fusion. The virus particle is uncoated upon gaining entry into the cell, and the genome is permitted to enter the cytoplasm. Coronavirus RNA acts as a messenger and is transported directly to the host cell Ribosomes. The host Ribosomes then replicate the RNA into RNA-dependent RNA polymerase (nsp12), RNA helicase (nsp13) and exoribonuclease (nsp14).

A number of the nonstructural proteins merge to form a multi-protein replicase-transcriptase complex. It is directly involved in the replication and transportation of RNA from an RNA strand. The replicase-transcriptase complex is also capable of genetic recombination when two viral genomes are present in the same infected cell. RNA recombination appears to be a significant driving force in determining genetic variability within coronavirus species. Coronavirus species' capability to jump from one host to another infrequently determines novel coronaviruses' emergence. The exact mechanism of recombination in coronaviruses is unclear but likely involves template switching during genome replication.

The replicated RNA becomes the new virus genome, and host ribosomes transform RNA into structural protein and ancillary protein. Viral structural proteins S, E and M migrate along the secretive pathway. M proteins direct most protein-protein interactions required for the assembly of viruses after binding to the nucleocapsids. The virus then spreads through secretive vesicles from the host cell by exocytosis. If the virus is released, it can infect other viruses. Coronavirus can cause the common cold and severe acute respiratory syndrome (SARS). The Middle East respiratory syndrome (MERS) and coronavirus disease in 2019 (COVID-19) are related to the same family.

The outbreak of COVID-19 was first identified in Wuhan, China, in December 2019. There are certain speculations that the virus was engineered by China to spread the virus and start a BioWare. Are those speculations true? What is the proof of those speculations? To explain that theory, I must explain to you what is an engineered virus and how are they made? Most importantly, how do we know if it is an engineered virus?

The engineered virus does not contain gears or, for that matter, any machine. An engineered virus is a genetically modified virus. A genetically modified virus is a virus that has been altered or generated using biotechnology methods and remains capable of infection. It includes directed insertion, deletion, artificial synthesis or change of nucleotide bases in viral genomes. It is not as easy as it may sound. It is made by inserting foreign genes into viral genomes. It is used for biomedical, agricultural, bio-control and technological objectives. In basic terms, the modification of RNA or DNA as per the specific needs of the virus is called a genetically modified virus.

Most DNA viruses have single monopartite genomes, and certain RNA viruses have multi-part genomes. Not all viral portions that are genetically engineered are considered to be genetically modified viruses. Viruses made from artificial gene synthesis are known to be genetically engineered viruses. Viruses that are only modified by random mutations or recombination.

Viruses are genetically modified to be used as a vector to insert or alter the genetic information into the host cell. Retroviruses are used for the genetically modified virus as they can genetically modify the host genes. So, the question arises, how are viruses genetically modified?

CRISPR does all the gene modification. It is also called Clustered Regularly Interspaced Short Palindromic Repeats. This program's basic principle is to remove or add a sequence of DNA or RNA in a virus, which then changes the organism's behaviour. It is used to locate the precise DNA sequence within the gene. An enzyme called Cas9 snips through the DNA, removing it or replacing it with a different set of DNA. It's used to replace a faulty gene with a healthy one or give it an upgrade.

CRISPR-C as a system is a prokaryotic immune system that confers resistance to foreign genetic elements such as those present within plasmids and phages and provides a form of acquired immunity. RNA harbouring the spacer sequence helps Cas (CRISPR-associated) proteins recognize and cut foreign pathogenic DNA. Other RNA-guided Cas proteins cut foreign RNA. CRISPR is found in approximately 50 per cent of sequenced bacterial genomes and nearly 90 per cent of sequenced archaea. This system has created CRISPR gene editing. This program has a wide range of applications.

The nuclease Cas12a (formerly known as Cpf1) was defined in CRISPR/Cpf1 in 2015. Cas12a revealed a variety of main variations between Cas9 and Cas12a.

It involves causing a 'staggered' cut in double-stranded DNA instead of a 'blunt' cut created by Cas9, depending on a 'T rich' PAM (providing alternate targeting sites to Cas9) requiring only a CRISPR RNA (crRNA) for effective targeting. The small CRNAs of Cas12a are suitable for multiplexed genome editing.

In 2016, the nuclease of the bacterium Leptotrichia shahi was characterized as Cas13a (formerly known as C2c2). Cas13 is an RNA-guided endonuclease, which means that it can only be bound to a single-stranded RNA. Its crRNA directs Cas13 to the target of the ssRNA. The distinguishing characteristic of Cas13, relative to Cas9, is that after the reduction of its target, Cas13 remains bound to its target. This property is called "collateral cleavage" and is used to establish various diagnostic technologies.

Before the upgrade is done to a virus, many genetic sequences or computer models run to predict the virus's behaviour. Most genetically modified viruses are used to treat cancer cells. A virus can be modified to attack a specific community, gene, colour, etc. There are many possibilities for it. A virus was modified in Germany that can affect the fertility of a woman. Once introduced in the environment, it can affect the foetus, which can cause miscarriages. Many might think that many have found a way to reduce the global population. But the problem is that if it affects 100 per cent of the population, then no one can give birth, eventually decreasing the world population, and it does not have a cure. There was a prediction made on the same model that since the virus affects the organism's genes, women might lose the ability to give birth.

An oncolytic virus is a genetically modified form of a herpesvirus for treating the melanoma that has been approved by the Food and Drug Administration (FDA). However, several viruses are being evaluated as potential treatments for cancer in clinical trials. When an oncolytic virus infects a host cell, they multiply and kill the cell. Once they multiply, they enter other cancer cells, and the cycle repeats. Their receptors are the same as the receptors on the cancer cells. They cannot harm a healthy cell.

CRISPR genetic modifications are used to treat or cause a pandemic. Once RNA or DNA is modified using CRISPR, it can be located in the later generations of the virus. These modifications are specific and just by analyzing the genetic sequence it can be identified if it is genitically modified manually or naturally. There is substancial proof that it is not genitically modified. A news report published by Medical News Today also proves that it is not human-made.

The new study appears in the journal Nature Medicine. Kristian Andersen, Ph.D, an associate professor of immunology and microbiology at the Scripps Research Institute in La Jolla, CA, is the first and corresponding author on the paper.

Andersen and colleagues set out to see what they could deduce from the study of available genomic evidence regarding the new coronavirus's origin. As the author states in their article, researchers have been attempting to locate the beginning of the pandemic of COVID-19.

Initially, experts linked the virus to a seafood market in Wuhan, China. At the same time, later study papers suggested that the virus may have spread to humans from illegally trafficked mammals called pangolins.

To evaluate the new virus's origin, the researchers compared the "backbone" of SARS-CoV-2 with other viruses that commonly affect bats and pangolins. They did so using genetic sequencing data that Chinese scientists made available.

Andersen and his team also looked at spike proteins that coronaviruses use to bind to the membranes of the human or animal cells they infect.

Ending the rumors about SARS-CoV-2

More specifically, the new research authors looked at two components of spike proteins: the receptor-binding domain (RBD), which latches onto healthy host cells, and the cleavage site, which opens up the virus and allows it to penetrate the host cell.

Spike proteins need a receptor on human cells called angiotensin-converting enzyme 2 (ACE2) to bind to human cells. The scientists found that the spike protein's receptor-binding domain had evolved to target ACE2 so effectively that it could only have been the result of natural selection and not of genetic engineering.

Furthermore, the molecular structure of the backbone of SARS-CoV-2 supported this finding. If scientists had engineered the new coronavirus as a pathogen, then the starting point would likely have been the backbone of another virus in the coronavirus family.

However, the backbone of SARS-CoV-2 was very different from those of other coronaviruses and was most similar to related viruses in bats and pangolins.

"These two features of the virus, the mutations in the RBD portion of the spike protein and its distinct backbone, rule out laboratory manipulation as a potential origin for SARS-CoV-2," explains Andersen.

Josie Golding, Ph.D., who is the epidemics lead at the Wellcome Trust, a research charity based in London, U.K., did not participate in the study but commented on its significance.

She says the findings are "crucially important to bring an evidence-based view to the rumours that have been circulating about the origins of the virus (SARS-CoV-2) causing COVID-19."

"[The authors] conclude that the virus is the product of natural evolution," Golding adds, "ending any speculation about deliberate genetic engineering." (Medical News Today)

This theory proves that we did not genetically modify the virus. But can it be spread intentionally? Well, it is a question that should be asked to the Chinese Government. But specific theories prove that detailed experiments were being conducted in Wuhan, China, and the virus was accidentally released from the lab. It is one of the theories which proved that 'patient zero' was a lab employee.

French Nobel prize-winning scientist Luc Montagnier has sparked fresh controversy by claiming that the SARS-CoV-2 virus came from a lab and resulted from an attempt to manufacture a vaccine against the AIDS virus. In an interview with French CNews channel and during a podcast by Pourquoi Docteur, professor Montagnier, who co-discovered HIV, claimed that there are strains of HIV and malaria in the coronavirus genome, according to a report in the Asia Times.

Forbes reported that "uncanny similarity of unique inserts in the 2019-nCoV spike protein to HIV-1 gp120 and Gag."

Based on the analysis of multiple, very short regions of proteins in the novel coronavirus, the bioRxiv paper claimed that the new coronavirus might have acquired these regions from HIV. Some types of viruses can swap pieces of their genetic code. In this case, the authors of the study say that the specific coronavirus involved in the most recent outbreak (2019-nCoV) has four small chunks of sequence in its genetic code that were not found in other, similar coronaviruses like SARS. According to the authors, these pieces bear some resemblance to bits of the sequence found in HIV.

It may not be a coincidence, and the pieces of genetic code may have been deliberately inserted there. The hypothesis that the novel coronavirus was developed and escaped from the Wuhan Institute of Virology at the advanced biocontainment facility of the Chinese Academy of Sciences. There is no explanation for the virus to have a genome sequence, and no other hypothesis explains that the genome was present. According to China Daily, all these arguments were nonsense.

Shi Zhengl said on social media on Sunday that the virus was the result of "nature punishing the uncivilized habits and customs of humans," and she is willing to "bet my life that the outbreak has nothing to do with the lab."

The best part of this hypothesis is that the same gene sequence could be present in certain other types of viruses but not in other coronaviruses. Finally, it was concluded that the virus had tiny segments of HIV-like protein that had no excuse to be present in coronavirus. Comparing the protein's small fragments, it is impossible to conclude if the virus was deliberately released. The report also tends to be false-positive.

The paper was finally withdrawn from bioRxiv on Sunday afternoon, with one of the authors state that: "It was not our intention to feed into the conspiracy theories, and no such claims are made here." The author further declares that the researchers will revise the paper and re-analyze the data before submitting it again.

Different countries had to deal with the pandemic differently. Many countries were on the verge of losing governance control. Some countries had to ask for help from different countries to get through the pandemic. Let's see how the virus spread through different countries and how it affects them.

According to some unpublished documents of the Chinese authorities, the first case can be dated back to 17 November 2019. He was a 55-year-old native of Hubei Province. Four men and five women reported being affected in November, but none of them were "patient zero." The World Health Organization's website notes that the first confirmed case of COVID-19 had occurred in China on 8 December. The WHO does not monitor the outbreak itself, and relies on nations to have the information. From November 17, a median of five cases a day was registered. Approximately, 27 patients were active cases by 15 December, and the cumulative number of active cases reached 60 by 20 December. After December 17, the first double-digit cases a day were reported.

In late December, Chinese doctors realized that they were dealing with a new type of infection. Until the Chinese doctors realized that they were dealing with some unknown disease, 266 people were infected. But they could not identify the patient zero, which is crucial for mapping wild animals' journeys to humans. Different reports from different countries have different theories of who "patient zero" is. It took years to find the first person who suffered from MERS, and it has never been fully established that SARS crossed the animal-human barrier.

Michael Ryan, the executive director of the WHO Health Emergencies Program, said that "patient zero could be outside China and that's why we have to keep an open-mind" Xinhua News Agency reported this. According to a study published by Chinese researchers in the Lancet medical journal on August 12th, 2020, the first person diagnosed by COVID-19 was on December 1, 2019. That person had "no contact" with the Huanan Seafood Wholesale Market, where the outbreak is thought to have first come to light. Many clues were used to track down patient zero, but many people already have positive antibodies in their bodies, making it difficult to identify an infection event.

Since March 30th, 2020, the Economic Times has indicated that the Wuhan prawn vendor is listed as "patient zero." The 57-year-old female prawn vendor in China's Wuhan City is recognized as the origin of the coronavirus pandemic. She was identified as one of the first victims of the coronavirus that has claimed almost 28,000 lives (at the time of the report). The coronavirus 'patient zero,' who recovered utterly in January after months of treatment, claims that the Chinese government might have managed to stop the disease's transmission if it had acted earlier.

As identified by The Wall Street Journal, Wei Guixian was selling prawns at the Seafood Market on December 10 when she developed a cold. Believing she had the common flu, she was given an injection for the flu. However, she continued to feel weak and visited Eleventh Hospital in Wuhan a day later. With the feeling of weakness, she visited one of the biggest medical facilities in Wuhan Union Hospital on December 16. At the Union Hospital, Wei was told that her sickness was "ruthless" and that many of Seafood Market had visited the hospital with matching symptoms.

At the end of December, Wei was quarantined when doctors related the coronavirus's emergence with the seafood market. The Mirror quoted a Chinese news outlet, The Paper, "Coronaviruses can cross species boundaries and adapt to new hosts, which allows us to predict more coronaviruses in the future more directly."

The article in The Paper concluded that the new coronavirus is likely to become the fifth endemic coronavirus in humans. Humans need more research to help formulate public health policies to deal with the emergence of similar viruses. So, the so-called "live market" has been closed indefinitely following the coronavirus outbreak.

Wei was one of the survivors and had regained her health in January. The COVID-19 'patient zero' believes she got the disease from a toilet she shared with the market's meat sellers. She said several vendors trading close to her also contracted the killer disease. In a release, the Wuhan Municipal Health Commission confirmed that Wei was among the first 27 patients to test positive for COVID-19 and one of 24 cases directly related to the market. Wei said the virus' death toll could have been lower if the government had "acted sooner."

Though identified as 'patient zero,' Wei may not be the first person to have contracted coronavirus in China, the report said.

– The Economic Times (March 30th, 2020)

Even after so many conspiracy theories, China has continued to fight the virus-like any other country. Not much was known about the infection, the cause, the effects and, most notably, the treatment. There was nothing more that could be done except treat the symptoms and hold the patient alive so that our bodies could recognize it and establish protection to it. Patients cannot be left open to relieve the symptoms since they can raise exposure chances. With the sudden increase in the number of infected people, there was a sudden increase in the need for managed hospital space. So, in 10 days, China constructed a temporary hospital, beginning work on 24 January.

On Sunday, the 2nd of February, China finished building an emergency hospital setup. They accepted the first patient on Monday, 3rd February. It is made up of two floors and is equipped with 1,000 beds, several isolation wards, and 30 intensive care units. China's health authorities said that 304 people had died from the coronavirus, with more than 14,000 cases in the country and beyond due to which they had to construct a hospital to control the infection. The entire facility was about 6,45,000 square feet.

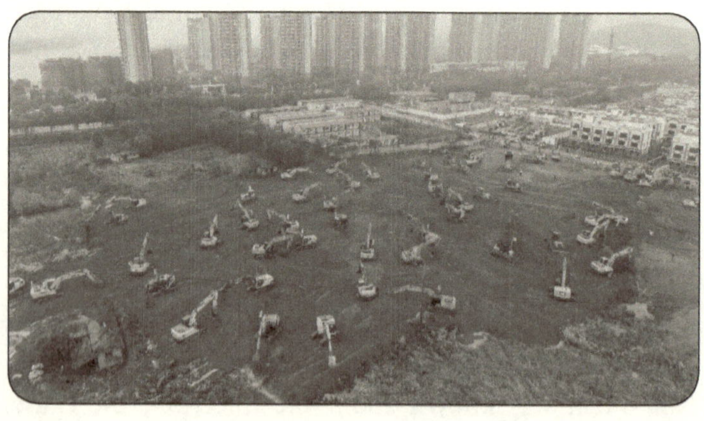

Excavator digging to level the land

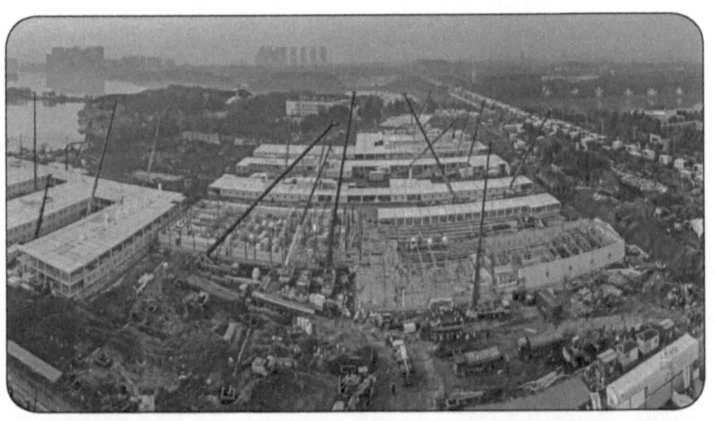

Truck pumping concrete

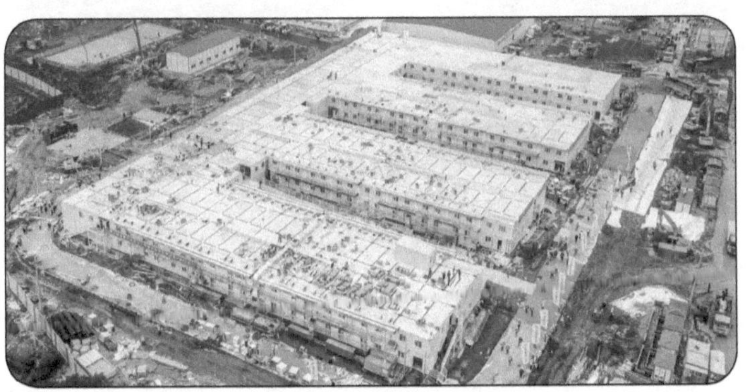

Hospital built and opened for business

But the question stands, how did they construct such a hospital in a matter of days?

Using prefabricated units is the key to constructing a building at such a fast speed. Instead of building the foundation and then following up the superstructure, prefabricated units allow the construction parallel.

Prefabricated units are like lego blocks. They both have male and female groves like the heart and soul in the lego parts. Prefabricated parts are built off the site in controlled conditions to achieve maximum strength at the highest efficiency at least cost.

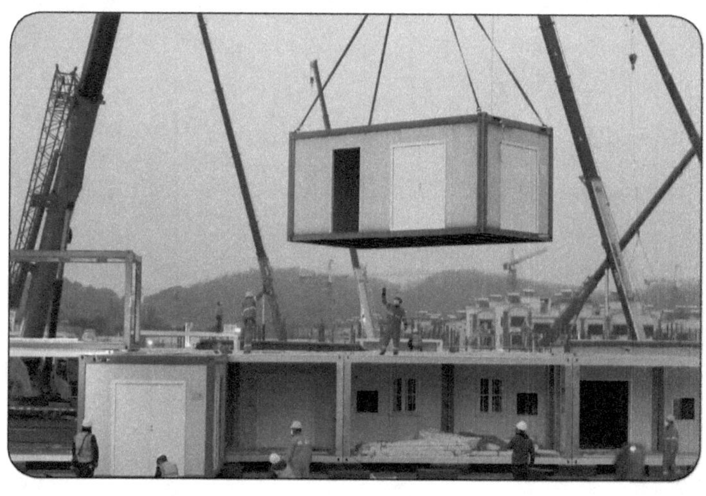

The prefabricated block being placed

The global architecture firm has designed dozens of hospitals and health care facilities around the world, including a design for Singapore's Community Hospital at Yishun (Singapore is one of the countries where people have been diagnosed with the virus). Since that's its only purpose, it is not a hospital in the conventional sense. This hospital has assessment and triage capabilities, some imaging capabilities, a clinical laboratory, a pharmacy and isolation rooms but not much else.

It's also important to distribute the air around the room in the right manner. Air must enter the room from the ceiling above the patient and must vary along the wall around the room's perimeter as air filtration is essential that use HEPA filtration. HEPA, which stands for High-Efficiency Particulate Air, refers to filtration that captures 99.97 per cent of the particles in the air passing through the filter. The same building was built in 2003, during SARS, which infected almost around 8,000 people and killed nearly 800 people. Xiaotangshan and Wuhan Huoshenshan Hospital is being built using prefabricated materials.

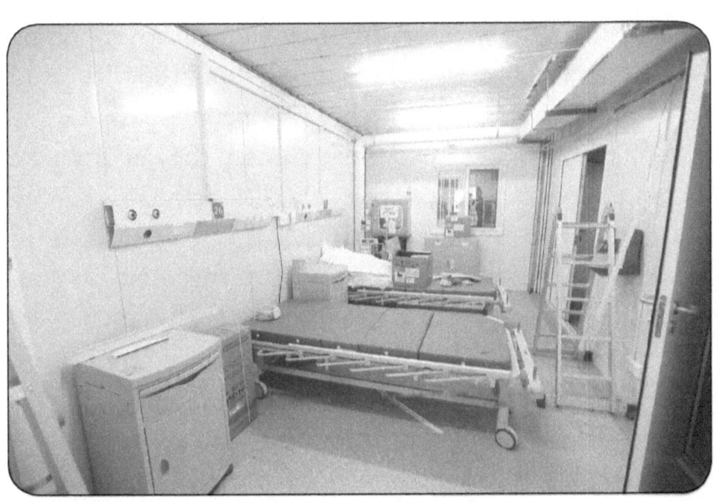

Beds inside the hospital

This same type of hospital was built during SARS in China. The major drawback of being in a country where the pandemic has started is that the government does not get a chance to control the pandemic. There is no data available about the pandemic that can be used to control it. No one knows how it affects, its symptoms and how it spreads. One of the best things about these projects is that the government or private companies did not fully control them. Bringing resources and knowledge together from the best companies is what kept the country running. Local people were also of great help where a lot of localities helped in the project. It is not just the output of knowledge and power but also the zeal to save the country. We can learn a thing or two from them to help develop our countries.

With all the support from all the countries, China has finally recovered. There were about 85,591 total cases in China, out of which 4,634 people passed away and 80,729 people recovered, having the fatality rate of about five per cent. There are 228 active cases, 227 patients are in mild condition and one patient is in critical condition. As of January 22, the total number of confirmed cases had reached 581 globally; there were 571 cases reported in China and 375 were reported in Hubei province. After many studies in the country said that it is human-to-human transmission, the Chinese authorities expanded its preventive measures. They announced a lockdown in Wuhan and Hubei province on January 24. All public transportation and airports were suspended to prevent everyone from leaving or entering. One day before the Spring Festival in China, this announcement was made to reduce the very high population movement, thus reducing the disease's spread.

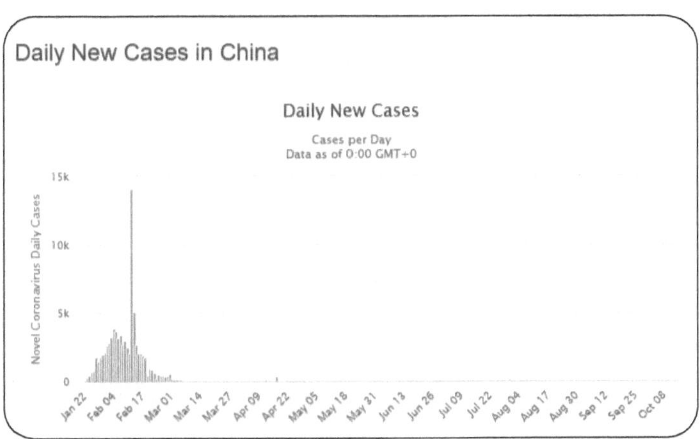

Many other countries had to suffer more than China. But why? Well, I would say it was their negligence. China had announced a lockdown to regulate the conditions where most countries were just getting up with the issues.

Thailand was the second country to report the first cases of COVID-19. The virus was confirmed to have reached Thailand on 13 January 2020, when the government made the first confirmation of China's claim. The number of cases was low throughout February, so they conducted a Muay Thai fight at the military-run Lumpinee Boxing Stadium on 6 March. Since then, the subjects increased by 100 per day, and the cases kept growing. Public venues and businesses were ordered to close in Bangkok and several other provinces, leading to the migration of people to their hometowns, so Prime Minister Prayut Chan-o-cha declared a state of emergency, effective on 26 March. The curfew has been in effect since 3 April.

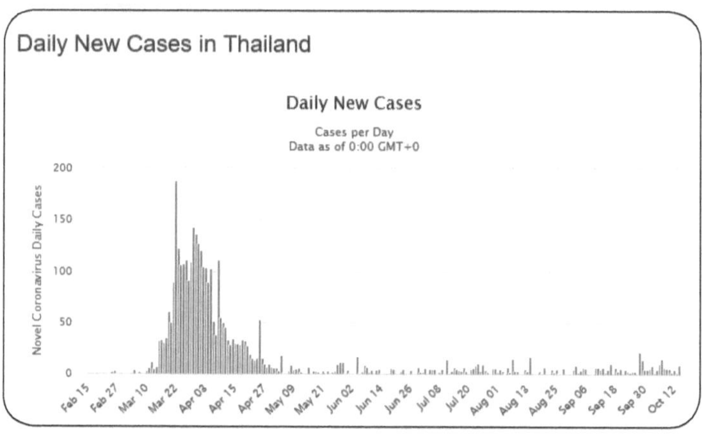

The varying lockdown protocol gradually controlled the cases, dropping the cases throughout April and May, and the rate of infection reached almost zero by the end of May. All commercial international flights were suspended from 4 April. Thailand had a total case of 3,665, of which 59 people passed away while 3,463 people have recovered to date. The public and country's robust public health infrastructure were credited as a combining factor for pandemic control's relative success. However, the state of emergency is still in effect in August.

It's estimated that Thailand's GDP will shrink by 6.7 per cent in 2020. The government had borrowed 1.9 trillion-baht (US$60 billion) for several assistance measures and cash handouts. But very few received it. Dissatisfaction with the government leads to the second wave of 2020. Thai protests starting on 18 July 2020.

The Thai Protest was the series of protests against Prayut Chan-o-cha, which have included demands for the Thai monarchy's reform. The protests were initially triggered by the dissolution of the Future Forward Party in late February 2020. The party was critical of Prayut and the country's political landscape, designed by the current 2017 constitution. This first wave of protests was held exclusively on academic campuses and was brought to a halt by the COVID-19 pandemic. The three demands for the rally were to dissolve parliament, to end intimidation of the people and to draft a new constitution. On 3 August, two student groups publicly raised demands to reform the monarchy. Ten demands for the reform of the monarchy were announced a week later. At the September 19 rally, 20,000–1,00,000 protesters were identified as an open challenge to King Vajiralongkorn. On 15 October, a "severe" state of emergency was declared in Bangkok, citing the royal motorcade's alleged blocking, which the authorities were accused of intentionally arranging through the rally site.

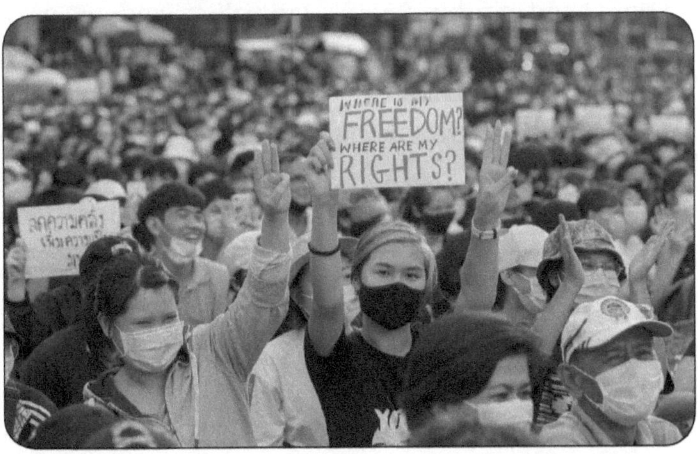

On July 15, the national centre of COVID-19 announced two new cases: an Egyptian soldier in Rayong

Province and a Sudanese diplomat's daughter in the Asok neighbourhood of Bangkok. Both of them were VIP guests and did not have to follow COVID regulations. Many criticized both the government's failure to contain the disease from those VIPs. This situation was considered the eruption point of the coming protest on 18 July.

❋ ❋ ❋

Japan was the third country to be hit by COVID-19. The Japanese government reported the first outbreak of the disease on 15 January 2020 in a Kanagawa Prefecture resident who had returned from Wuhan, China. On 30 January, Prime Minister Shinzo Abe established the Japan Anti-Coronavirus National Task Force to adapt, measure and control the outbreak. Japan is known to have the lowest death rate despite its ageing population. Cultural habits such as bowing etiquette, wearing face masks, hand washing with sanitizing equipment, a protective genetic trait and a relative immunity conferred by the mandatory BCG tuberculosis vaccine are some of the reasons they have the least death rate. Japan had two waves of COVID-19. The National Institute of Infectious Diseases has determined from its genetic research that the COVID-19 variant was two types.

The first wave was derived from the Wuhan type prevalent in patients from China and East Asia. It was followed by the second wave, which had its origin from France, Italy, Sweden and the United Kingdom. Japanese medical surveillance observed a second wave on 26 March, when the government advisory panel concluded that travellers and returnees from Europe and the United States were likely to cause a new outbreak between 11 March and 23 March. Data on the cases strongly suggest that Japan had successfully contained the Wuhan variant, and the European variant was spreading across the country. Therefore, there has been a spike in cases since the 26th of June. In terms of the number of confirmed COVID-19 cases, Japan overtook China on 5 October. Japan had a total active case of 90,104 with total casualties of 1638, and 83,158 people had recovered with a total death rate of two per cent to date.

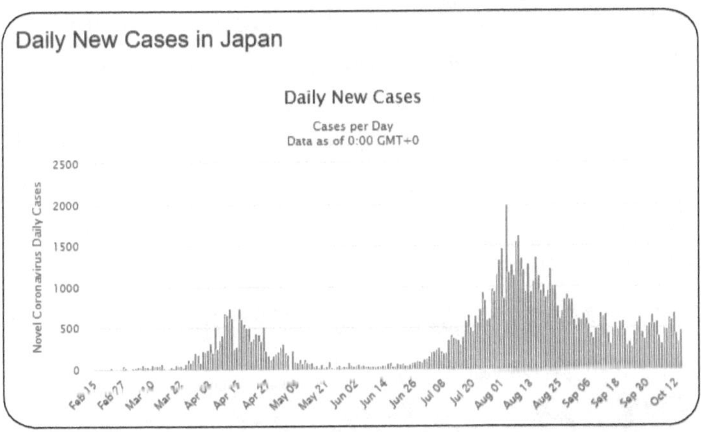

Japan now ranks 48 in the world in terms of total cases. Mr Abe, the Prime Minister of Japan, had finally declared an emergency on April 7. As businesses were closed, schools and nurseries were shut and people were self-isolated, anxious humanity awaited for the details of the government's plan to tackle the crisis. To fight the crises, Abe had started 'Abenomasks' for every house. Masks were posted to every home in Japan. But, that's remembered as an ineffectual waste of taxpayer's money.

Once the masks began to be delivered, there were further complaints of the products being stained, damaged or contaminated with human hair and dust. A large number had to be recalled.

Abe had addressed the people through a video to persuade the nation about the small pleasures of staying at home. It featured the PM cuddling his dog in his spacious apartment, winding down with a large, presumably warm beverage and watching TV. Simultaneously, most of the Japanese lived in cramped accommodations struggling to live by the day in uncertain economic conditions. Osaka's governor was pleading for raincoat donations since doctors had to wear trash bags as protective gear. A tweeter responds to the situation: "When so many people seem sluggish to strangle (with the virus), you look so elegant." Why don't you go and see hospitals that have been the battleground?"

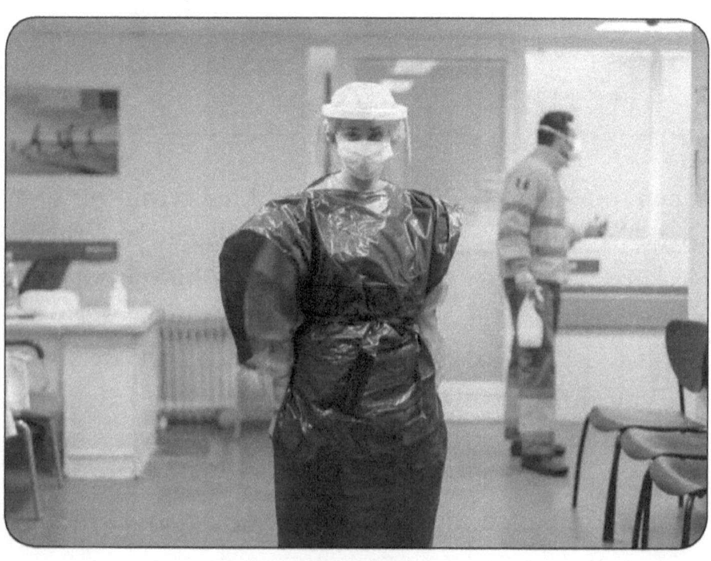

Ichiro Matsui, the mayor of Osaka, suggested that women stay at home and send men to do the grocery shopping instead since men were more directed and less likely to dawdle in shops. Speaking to reporters, he said, "Women take a long time as they browse around and hesitate about this and that," adding, "Men can snap up things they are told (to buy) and go, so I think it's good that they go shopping." Social media was once again less than appreciative. A tweeter had tweeted, "When I hear remarks like this. I feel the need for people with diverse backgrounds to participate in politics." More was expected from the leader than sops in the form of masks or feel-good videos about cuddling pets.

The pandemic has led India and the U.S. to suffer the most. They are also countries where COVID-19 patients are ranked highest. More than 79,00,000 cases and 2,16,000 COVID-19 deaths occurred in the U.S. in October 2020, accounted for 20 per cent of the COVID-19 casualties in the world. COVID-19 incidents in the U.S. gross 82,06,034, restoring a gross of 2,22,633 and 53,08,029 victims. In America, 26,75,372 are complete active events. The first case identified in the United States was on 20 January, and on 31 January, the epidemic was legally an emergency in public health. Many flights arriving from China were restricted. But the initial reaction was slow in planning healthcare, checking for viruses and avoiding other trips.

All 50 countries had confirmed cases by the end of March. Government and state reactions to the pandemic entail probation and cancellation of large-scale celebrations, such as concerts and athletic activities, school closures and homestays that facilitate study. All travel restrictions were extended to and from China on 2 February. Full limitations on travel have been applied in some countries, such as 14 days of quarantine and health inspections. On February 25, for the first time, the U.S. population was alerted to brace for a local epidemic by the Centers for Disease Control and Prevention (CDC). They were asked to take care without any vaccination or medication.

In the meantime, pandemic limitations have been implemented. By March 12, the number of cases diagnosed with COVID-19 in the U.S. surpassed 1,000. On 13 March, travel bans were applied to and from European countries. Several states were required to remain home with quarantine throughout March and April to monitor the virus's transmission. By the end of March 27, more than 1,00,000 cases had been registered by the country. On April 2, at President Trump's direction, the Centers for Medicare & Medicaid Services (CMS) and CDC ordered additional preventive guidelines requiring temperature checks for anyone in a nursing home, symptom screenings, and requiring all nursing home personnel to wear face masks. Trump also said COVID-19 patients should have their buildings or units and dedicated staffing teams. On April 11, the U.S. death toll became the highest since the number of deaths reached 20,000, surpassing Italy's.

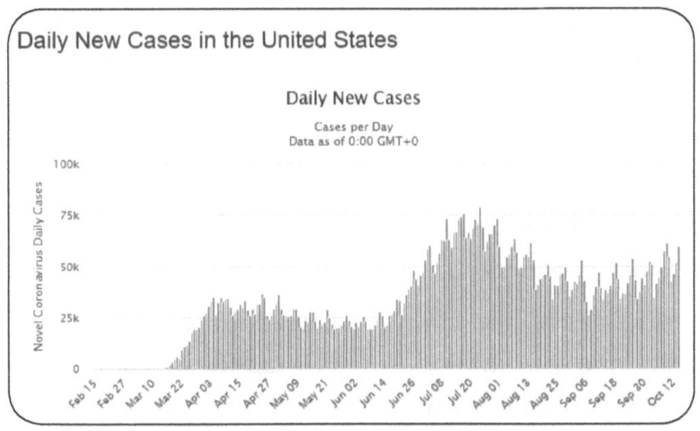

In July, the U.S. recorded the highest number of cases per day globally, with 77,638 patients per day. President Trump wore a protective mask for the first time on July 11. On October 2, 2020, Trump announced on Twitter that both he and the First Lady had tested positive for the coronavirus and would immediately quarantine, resulting in several White House staff and contacts testing positive. Does the question arise, what will happen if the president passes away? Who will take over the country's roles? The Deputy Chief of the Coast Guard, Charles W. Ray, also tested positive for COVID-19. Other military officials were quarantined.

The cases of COVID-19 are moderate and are estimated to be restored quickly enough. Presidents dying in the line of work were quite rare. Unfortunately, the country has quite a bit of history in presidents' deaths, with eight dying in office, from William Henry Harrison in 1841 to John F. Kennedy in 1963. As revised and augmented by revisions and constitutional enactments, the Constitution provided that the Vice-President shall hold the highest office automatically after the President's deaths. In the same situation, if anything happens to the Vice-President, the next speaker will be in the line of succession, and then the President will be in the House. The twenty-fifth amendment, passed in 1967, lays out a procedure for replacing the Vice-President after he or she becomes President.

In March, the country had about 12 million N95 masks and 30 million surgical masks in the Strategic National Stockpile, but only roughly 1.2 per cent of the approximately 3.5 billion masks required. As of March, there were 19,000 ventilators available, out of which 16,660 were immediately available and 2,425 were in maintenance. By the end of March, hundreds of tonnes of medical-grade face masks were shipped by air freight to foreign buyers in China and other countries. In August 2020, supply problems persisted when a survey reported that 42 per cent of nurses experienced widespread or intermittent personal protective equipment shortages, with 60 per cent using single-use equipment for five or more days.

An unexpectedly high percentage of COVID-19 patients (about 20 per cent) in the ICU required dialysis due to kidney failure. In mid-April, workers at several hospitals in New York City reported not having enough dialysis equipment and running low on fluids to operate machines. They reported a shortage of dialysis nurses, as many were ill with COVID-19 due to a lack of adequate PPE. President Trump has denied the PPE shortages, calling them "fake news." In September, he quoted, "We've opened up factories; we've had tremendous success with face masks and with shields." As per individual sources who work in medical facilities, they were not given appropriate PPE kits, including the whole set of masks, screens, gloves, protective overcoat and glasses. Sometimes, they had to wear the same set for a couple of days, which were no longer sterile.

❋ ❋ ❋

India ranks second in the total number of reported cases in the world. India has a total of 73,70,468 COVID-19 cases with casualties of 1,12,161, and 64,48,658 people had recovered. The first case of COVID-19 had originated from China on 30 January 2020. India has the largest number of confirmed cases in Asia. India currently holds the single-day record for the most massive increase in cases, set on September 17, with an additional 97,894. The rate of fatalities in India is among the lowest in the world at about 2 per cent. By mid-May 2020, six cities accounted for around half of all reported cases in the country – Mumbai, Delhi, Ahmedabad, Chennai, Pune, and Kolkata. As of 10 September 2020, Lakshadweep is the only region that has not reported a case.

On 22 March, Prime Minister Narendra Modi declared a voluntary public curfew, accompanied by a 21-day national lockdown on 24 March, accompanied by a sporadic extension of the lockdown and a final lockdown on 1 June. After the lockdown in March, the United Nations (UN) and the World Health Organisation (WHO) lauded India's response as 'comprehensive and rigorous,' calling the lockdown restrictions 'aggressive but essential' to curb the spread and develop the requisite healthcare infrastructure. In June, India was ranked

56th out of 200 countries in the Deep Information Group's protection assessment survey COVID-19.

The first fatality recorded on March 12th in India was a 76-year-old man with a travel history to Saudi Arabia. A Sikh preacher, who travelled to Italy and Germany, turned into a "super spreader" by attending a Sikh festival in Anandpur Sahib during 10–12 March. 27 COVID-19 cases were traced back to him. Over 40,000 people in 20 villages in Punjab were quarantined on 27 March to contain the spread. On 31 March, a Tablighi Jamaat religious congregation event in Delhi, which took place earlier in March, emerged as a new virus super spreader after numerous cases across the country were traced back to it. On 18 April, the Health Ministry announced that 4,291 cases were directly linked to the event. On 2 May in Punjab, around 4,000 stranded pilgrims returned from Hazur Sahib in Nanded, Maharashtra. Many of them tested positive, including 27 bus drivers and conductors who had been part of the transport arrangement. As of 13 May, 1,225 pilgrims had been tested positive.

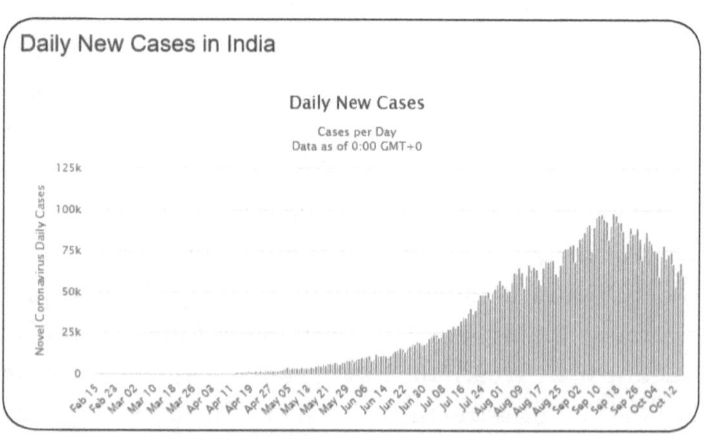

On 16 April, 6,50,000 rapid antibody and RNA extraction kits were shipped from China, and more than 2 million kits were shipped in the next 15 days. On 21 April, the West Bengal Ministry of Health reported that many of the test kits supplied by ICMR-NICED had yielded inconclusive results. Rapid antibody studies were supposed to have 90 per cent precision, although the studies' real accuracy was 5.4 per cent. Later, the ICMR told all states to avoid using kits for two days. Lastly, it was put on hold until further notice.

Chinese manufacturers of rapid and RNA extraction kits said that the ICMR accepted the test kits, and the issue was how the kits were used and not the kits themselves. However, they have agreed to cooperate with the Indian authorities to resolve this problem. Later, ICMR ordered that the kits be returned to the Chinese retailer, and the order was cancelled.

I have visited ten hospitals, and only two hospitals provided all the resources, making it only 20 per cent of the hospitals. The remaining 80 per cent of hospitals had to recycle their resources or provide just some basic protection kit. Some hospitals could not even start accepting the patients as the government did not allow them due to unavailable resources. It means the employees of the hospitals lost their jobs and had to search for another hospital. It reduced the capacity of the hospitals. The government took specific steps to help hospitals reinstate, like supplying PPE kits, ventilators and other sanitization equipment.

I have a friend who is a nurse at Breach Candy Hospital. Her name is Shirin Joseph Vadakkan. She works hand in hand with COVID-19 patients. I interviewed her to learn more about how the hospital copes with the growing cases and how it handles cases. Let me start by telling you more about the hospital. Breach Candy ranks 17 in Mumbai. Breach Candy Hospital is a private hospital located in Mumbai, India. The hospital has a patient to nurse ratio of 1:1. Since Shirin is a nurse, she has to stay in touch with the patients continually. As the lockdown began, she was given 15 days of holiday. Initially, not all hospitals were equipped to handle COVID-19 patients, and on the other hand, due to lack of transport, the hospital was running on a limited staff. When her holiday ended, they were educated about the PPE suit and the hospital's emergency protocol regulations.

Due to the pandemic, several emergency procedures have been modified. They were supplied with a new PPE kit every day. Their apparel consisted of three layers of protection. When they enter the hospital, they have a full-body bath with disinfectant soap and wear a scrub like they usually have. She's working in the ICU, so her scrub is green in colour. She's wearing a gown over the scrub, followed by a PPE kit. You can see a girl in green scrub with an N95 mask and slippers. Her kit consists of surgical gloves, surgical masks and surgical headgear along with scrub and gown. The entire collection is known to be 'two levels of defence.' Overall, they wear a PPE pack, which includes a gown, a pair of governors, headgear, shades, a couple of shoe covers, and an N95 mask. Initially, all the PPE kits were made of plastic that suffocated them. Later, it was changed to a fabric-based PPE pack.

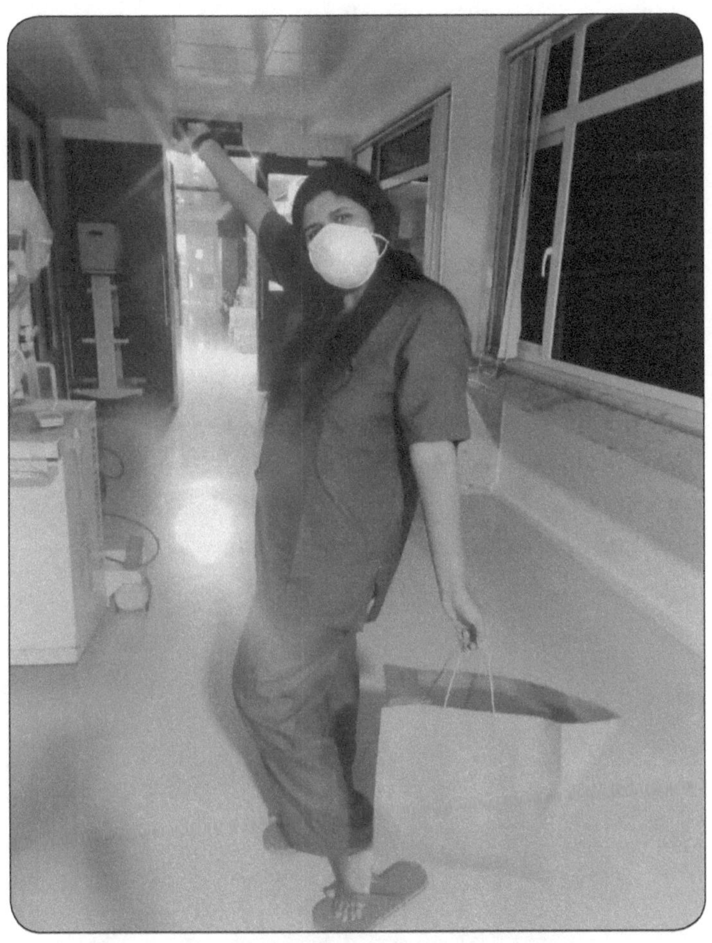

Shirin is wearing her srub along with an N95 mask after her shift. Due to the lockdown, they did not have any transportation mode, so the hospital provided them with food and shelter for the meantime. They used to stay in hospital hostels and had food in the hospital cafeteria.

Once they are up in their protective kits, they are given Hydroxychloroquine. This medicine can kill an

RNA-based virus. This medicine is used to prevent and treat malaria in areas where malaria remains sensitive to chloroquine. Other uses include the treatment of rheumatoid arthritis, lupus and porphyria cutanea tarda. It is prescribed periodically by the doctors. When they take it for the first time, they have to take two tablets, and later, it is prescribed every three to four days by the doctors. All the nurses dedicated to COVID-19 work in pairs. Only a nurse with a full PPE kit can handle COVID-19 patients. While a nurse with a PPE kit takes care of the patient, the other nurse keeps tabs on the forms and other entries or documents necessary for the patient. They have a shift of 12 hours, and they wear the PPE kit for about 6 hours each.

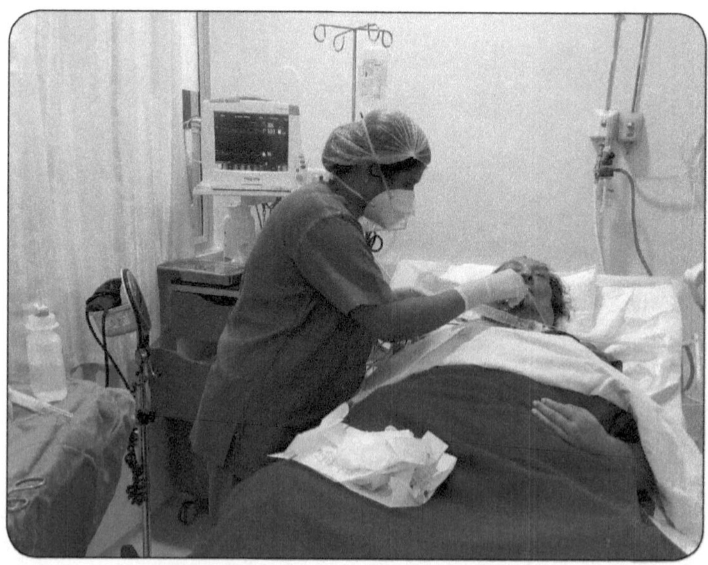

The nurse is wearing her scrub along with a mask and a headgear during her shift and treating a non-COVID-19

patient. Gloves, masks and headgear were mandatory for everyone.

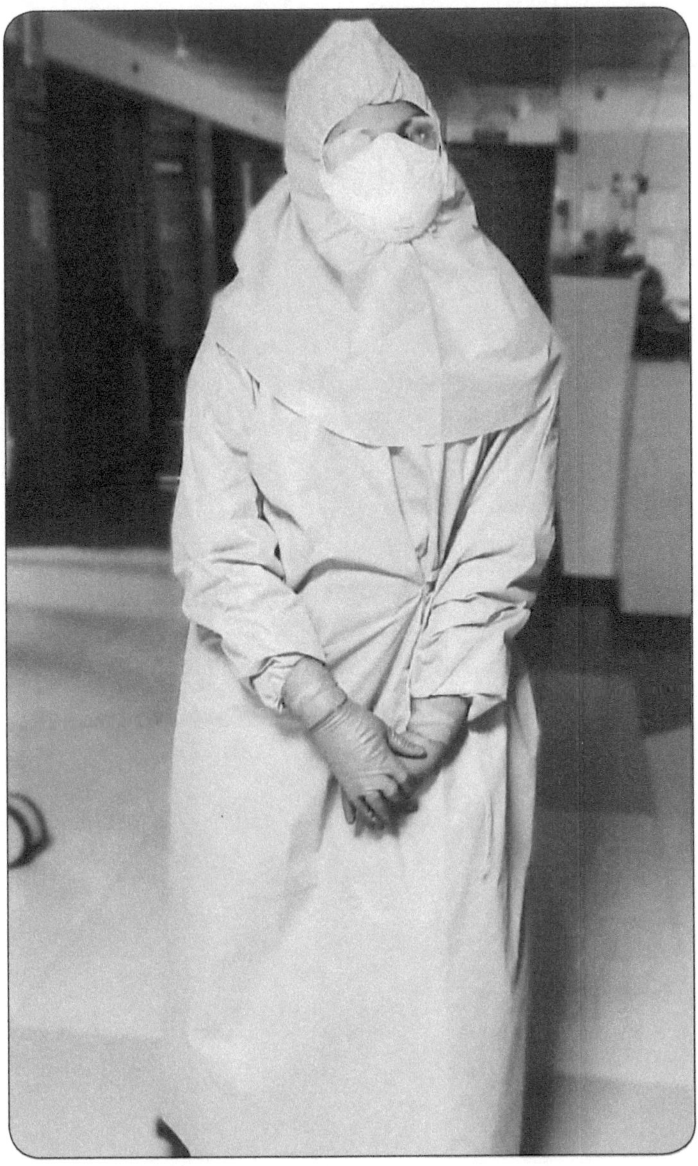

Shirin is wearing her full PPE kit during her shift to work with COVID-19 patients. PPE kit was compulsory to treat COVID-19 patients.

Once they're done with their shift, they've got to have a full-body bath, and the PPE kit is disposed off. Their dress and scrub are all put in a laundry room for cleaning, and they are not allowed to take their clothes home as there is a risk of infection. As a token of their hard work and compassion, they were given a raise of 50 per cent, and if they die because of COVID-19, their family will be given Rs 33 Lakhs each. That's the money the hospital has to sell. All the additional costs of PPE kits, other wearables, food and nurses' stay were additional costs added to the billings. Not every patient can afford to pay, and not every hospital can offer it.

Every country had to deal with the pandemic differently depending on their financial condition and the policies. On the other hand, every country played a different political role. So, is there a cure for the pandemic? Will there ever be? Let me take you to the next chapter, "The Cure."

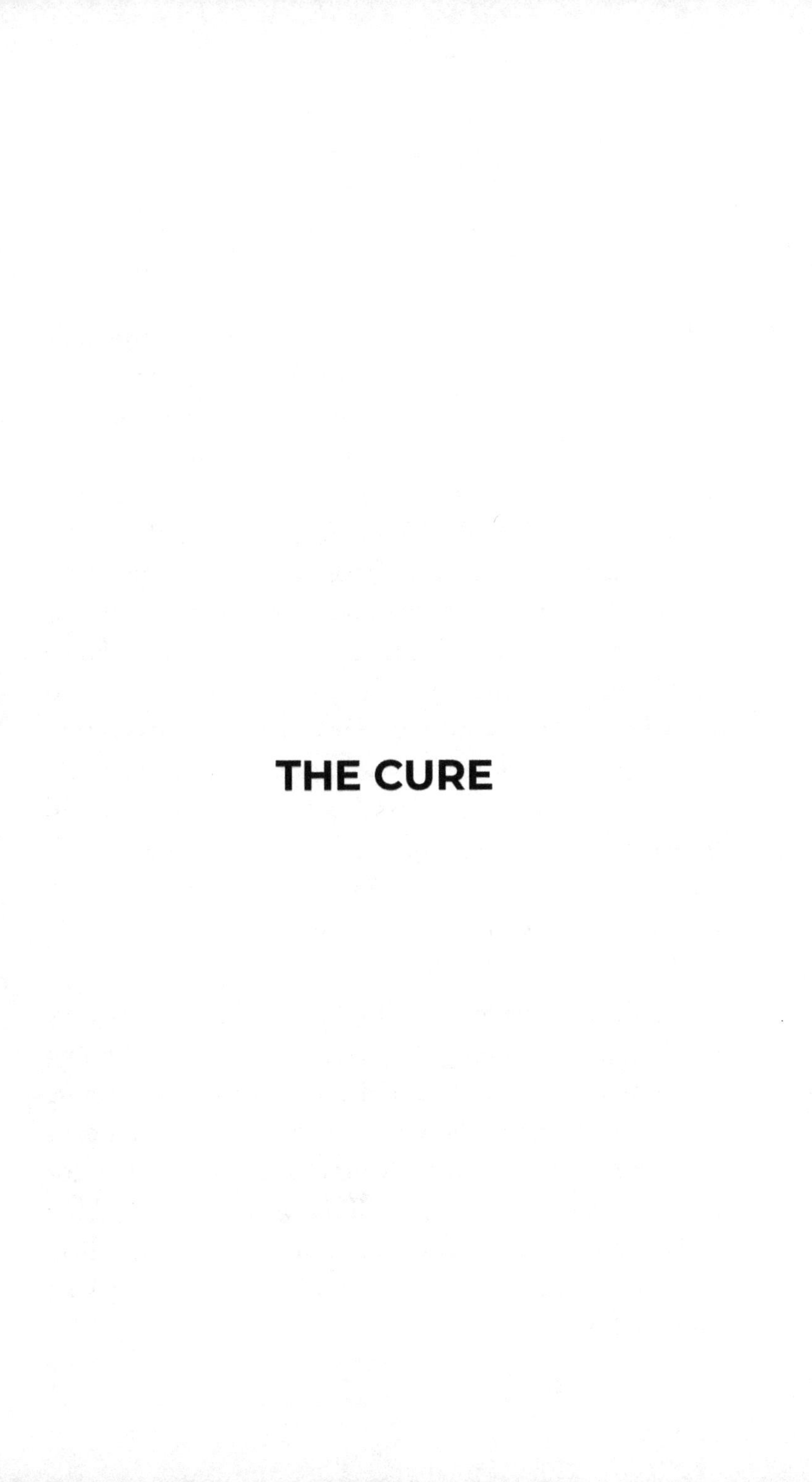

THE CURE

To get into the cure, we need to understand how the virus affects our bodies. What are the crucial organs it affects, and what are the consequences of the virus's effects? Other than just infecting the host, some consequences are fatal for us. The most common symptoms of COVID-19 are fever, tiredness and dry cough. Some patients may have aches and pains, nasal congestion, runny nose, sore throat or diarrhoea. These symptoms are usually mild and begin gradually. Some people get sick but don't develop any symptoms and don't feel ill. About 80 per cent of people recover from the illness without needing extra care. 1 out of every six people who have COVID-19 become critically ill and have trouble breathing. Aged individuals, including those with chronic medical conditions such as elevated blood pressure, respiratory problems or diabetes, are most likely to experience serious illnesses.

It all happens as the infection reaches the body by inhaling air containing droplets and viruses or rubbing the contaminated surface and then touching your nose or mouth. It offers the virus a path across the mucous membranes of the throat. It may take 2 to 14 days for the virus to show symptoms. If the virus has entered the body, it infects the organs by entering healthy cells. There the invader makes clones of himself and multiplies all over the body.

The new coronavirus (COVID-19) latches its spiky surface proteins to receptors on healthy cells, especially those in your lungs. Specifically, viral proteins bust into cells through ACE2 receptors. Once inside, the coronavirus hijacks healthy cells and takes command. Eventually, it kills some of the healthy cells. Some of them leave a genetic marker on the healthy cell, which can later on multiply. It is like adding its genome to the host healthy cell gene, which can replicate when the cell is about to die. When the host cell replicates, the viral gene will also replicate. That is one of the reasons that makes the virus more deadly. The virus moves down your respiratory tract. That's the airway that includes your mouth, nose, throat and lungs. Your lower airways, like alveoli, have more ACE2 receptors than the rest of your respiratory tract. So, COVID-19 is more likely to get darker than viruses like the common cold. The lungs can become inflamed, making it difficult for you to breathe. It can lead to pneumonia, an inflammation of tiny airbags (called alveoli) within the lungs, where the blood exchanges oxygen and carbon dioxide.

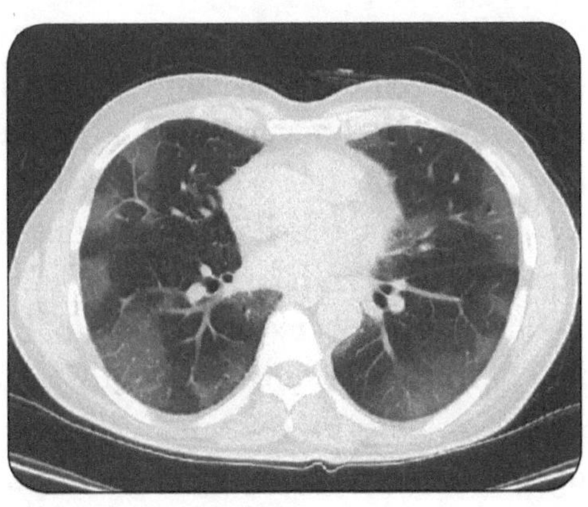

The above image shows the CT scan of the lungs with clouded regions due to COVID-19 infection.

In most people, the symptoms end with cough and fever. More than eight out of the 10 cases are moderate. But for others, the infection is getting more severe. There was shortness of breath around five to eight days after symptoms began (known as dysponea). A few days later, acute respiratory distress syndrome (ARDS) begins.

As the air sacs cannot transfer oxygen to the blood, the blood goes to a hypoxic state. Hypoxia is a state when the blood's deprived of oxygen, which reduces protein S, a natural anticoagulant. Due to the reduction in the levels of anticoagulant, the blood cells form clusters and clots. Clots can cause deep vein thrombosis, peripheral artery disease, atherosclerosis, etc. All clots can lead to heart attacks, organ failure, or the clot can also travel to the brain, causing some deadly damage, which can be fatal or cause some severe damage.

As it usually takes 2–14 days for the body to produce antibodies to destroy the virus, the doctors had to keep the patient alive by ensuring that adequate oxygen is supplied to the body. When the patient becomes so severe, they are attached to the ventilator so that the pressure on the lungs reduces, and the body receives adequate oxygen. Also, a ventilator might not be necessary if a person is fit with no pre-existing medical conditions. Only the right treatment will be enough. However, patients with pre-existing health problems are likely to be affected as their body will not combat the virus as it should, will hinder the healing process and will raise the life-threatening risk. For a person who is tested positive and treated appropriately to prevent clots, blood thinners are administered. But if COVID-19 was not identified and was treated automatically, then blood clots can form but cannot be located. In those cases, the patient might die of a heart attack, and the patient might not be aware that it was due to COVID-19. It will be a case of a normal heart attack. That is one reason why we might hear about a lot of deaths caused due to heart attacks.

So, how do we know if a person has COVID-19? There are two types of tests: detecting the antibody and detecting the infection itself. During the tests, blood is drawn, and antibody tests are conducted. These tests are designed to catch those antibodies and indicate whether someone has had COVID-19 in the past. However, such tests aren't always accurate, and antibodies can gradually disappear from someone's blood over time. When testing COVID-19, small antigen proteins from the SARS-CoV-2 virus are coated on a tray. They are then exposed to the patient's blood serum, where an enzyme and a chemical reagent are used. If the unique antibodies attacking the SARS-CoV-2 virus are found in the bloodstream, they would be bound to the viral antigen marker.

The enzyme then sticks to the antibody, which activates the chemical reagent, causing a colour change or giving off luminescence, indicating a positive result. Are all of the tests 100 per cent accurate? No, the tests aren't 100 per cent true, even in controlled laboratory conditions. But they are considered conclusive. The problem with these tests is that if you are infected and your body has still not detected the virus, then it will not create any antibodies, and the test will be negative, proving that you don't have COVID-19. These tests are relatively cheaper than other tests that use the virus or infection, causing organisms. So, to have more conclusive results, we have to test the infection-causing organism or virus itself. Those tests were conducted using Polymerase Chain Reaction (PCR).

Polymerase Chain Reaction (PCR) is a mechanism that amplifies (replicates) a small, well-defined fragment of DNA hundreds of thousands of times, generating enough of it for study. Certain kinds of chemicals were added to the sample to separate the DNA and RNA. Reverse transcription translates RNA to DNA. The method is called Reverse Transcription Polymerase Chain Reaction. It is a process used to transform RNA into DNA and, a polymerase chain reaction is used to amplify DNA. Coronavirus is an RNA virus, so this method is used to identify this type of virus. It takes a couple of hours to complete the process and is one of the most favoured methods. The technique can be streamlined with the appropriate equipment.

Samples can be obtained for examination using a combination of nasopharyngeal swabs, sputum (coughed up material), throat swabs, in-depth airway material obtained by a suction catheter, or saliva. For the COVID-19, most of the samples are collected from nasal, and throat swabs are collected. From a medical perspective, it is essential to remember that nasal and throat swabs tend to be less appropriate for diagnosis. These materials contain considerably less viral RNA than sputum, and the virus may escape detection if only these materials are tested. The sample needs to be collected from the alveoli to have the best test possible. As alveoli have mostly ACE2 receptors, and COVID-19 virus binds to the same receptors. But this is the best sample we can get. The cost of Reverse Transcription Polymerase Chain Reaction can cost around INR 2,500 to 10,000.

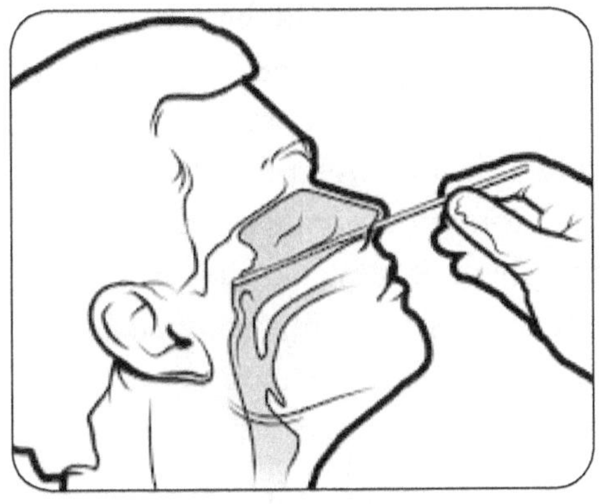

The image shows the extraction of the sample from a nasopharyngeal swab.

Antigen tests can be conducted on the spot. Antigen tests look for antigen proteins on the virus' surface. In the case of coronavirus, these are usually surface spike proteins. They're sort of a fast test, but they're not as reliable as the PCR tests. Samples can be obtained from a nasopharyngeal swab or saliva and are then exposed to strips of paper containing artificial antibodies meant to bind to coronavirus antigens. Antigens connect to the strips and provide visual reading. The procedure takes less than 30 minutes and will yield outcomes at the treatment point. It does not require costly equipment or intensive preparation. These tests might not be as conclusive as RT-PCR, but it can be a necessary test to be connected when the number of tests was required to conduct. These rapid tests do not require any form of training or fancy equipment. At the same time, RT-PCR requires a specific type of training. So, the question arises, if an infection is detected, is there a medicine available for it?

Viruses are tough to kill because they are organic matter with some genetic code but do not have any cell wall like bacteria or any other cell. They require a specific set of receptors to identify and kill them. They replicate rapidly. With every new organism, they tend to take over; they modify their genes, and the outcomes stand that modern medicine is probably required to kill the virus. But many drugs are in development. SARS-CoV and MERS-CoV still do not have a cure.

Many clinical trials are underway to explore treatments used for other conditions that could fight COVID-19 and develop new ones. People who are in the hospital with severe COVID-19 may get an antiviral medicine called redeliver. Research shows that some patients recover faster after taking it. Remdesivir was created to fight Ebola, but the FDA has issued an emergency use ruling so doctors can use it against COVID-19. Clinical trials are underway for other medications, including tocilizumab, which has been used to treat autoimmune conditions and an inflammatory condition called cytokine release syndrome.

The FDA has also approved an emergency authorization to use hydroxychloroquine and chloroquine to treat people hospitalized with COVID-19 amid serious concerns about their safety and how well they worked against the virus. These medications were used to treat malaria and autoimmune conditions. Studies have found that dexamethasone, a common steroid medication, can help people hospitalized with severe COVID-19 complications. But the findings are preliminary, and the researchers haven't released the full study.

One of the approaches used to treat COVID-19 is plasma transfusion. It is also called transfusion of blood plasmas. This procedure is officially a FDA approved procedure that is used to treat several patients. When a patient is sick, their bodies produce antibodies to kill the virus. These antibodies are found in the blood plasma. The plasma can be separated from the blood and administered to the patient. The patient's body recognizes that antigens are beginning to multiply. The problem with this theory is that there is not enough plasma to be administered to anyone. There are many drug experiments on the way.

Solidarity is a medicine developed by the World Health Organization and its partners to treat COVID-19 effectively. On 4th July, the WHO accepted the recommendation from the Solidarity Trial's International Steering Committee to discontinue the trial's hydroxychloroquine and lopinavir/ritonavir arms. The drug is still in medical trials and is under monitoring by 12,000 patients in over 500 hospitals in 30 countries. It is used to evaluate three different outcomes: mortality, need for ventilation and hospital stay-in days until there is sufficient evidence that the drug can be a potential cure without significant side effects. The WHO cautions against using medicine for medical and self-medication use. The Solidarity Trial published interim results on 15 October 2020. It found that all four treatments evaluated (redeliver, hydroxychloroquine, lopinavir/ritonavir and interferon) had little or no effect on overall mortality, initiation of ventilation and duration of hospital stay in hospitalized patients. Like every virus Covid-19 is also a virus and can mutate. If the virus mutates, the antigens in the body might not be as effective. The same thing goes on with the cure developed for the Coronavirus. Every country had to deal with the pandemic differently depending on their financial condition and the policies. Let's see some countries that handled things differently and have achieved something great. Let's start with the safest country to visit.

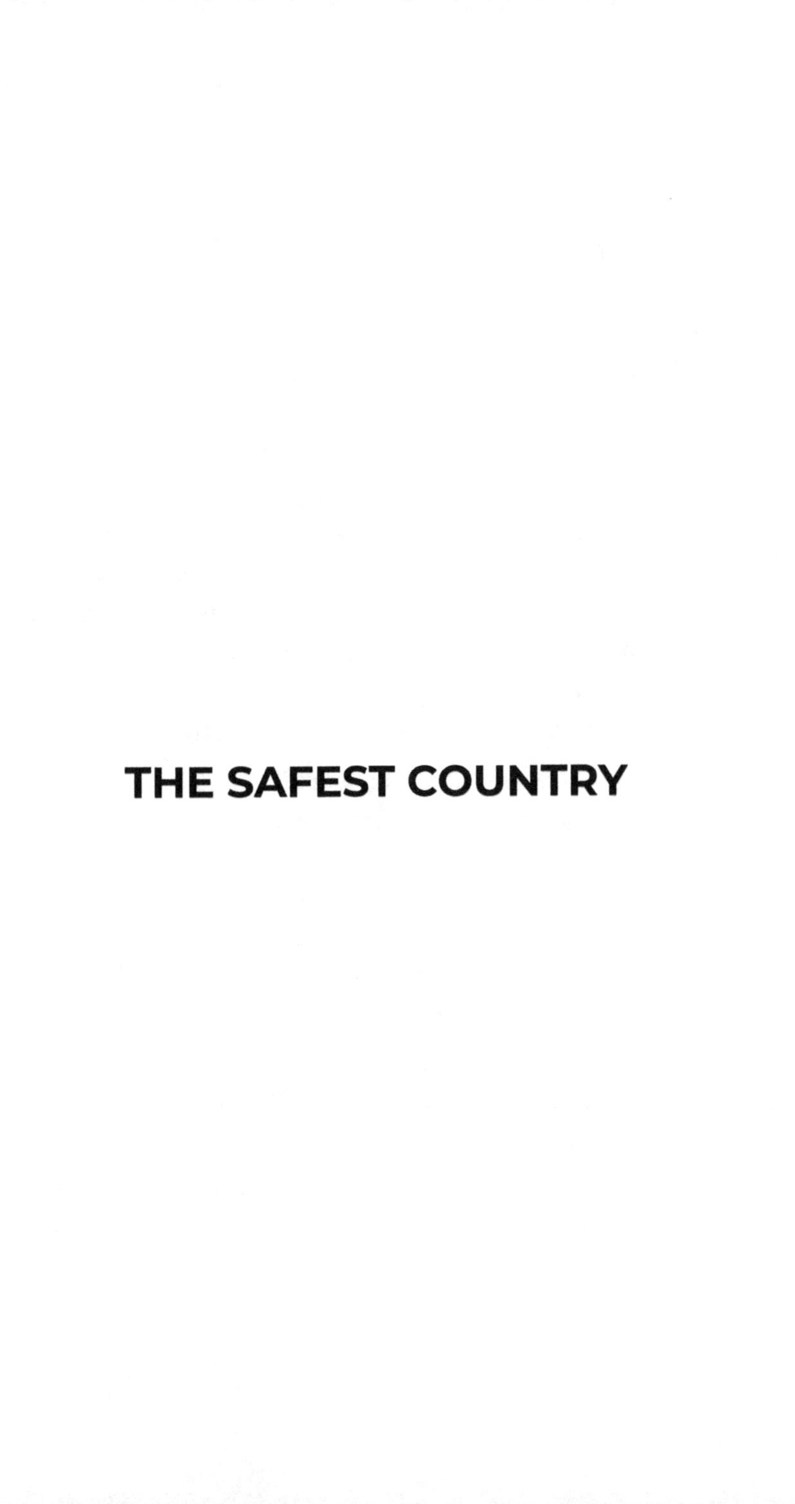

THE SAFEST COUNTRY

A study by the Deep Knowledge Group had conducted an analysis based on several factors that affect the COVID-19. The rankings were decided based on a total score of 752 points against all 130 parameters under categories of quarantine efficiency, healthcare readiness and risk management among others. As of August 2020, here is the list of countries that are considered safe. Switzerland was rated at the top of the list, followed by Germany and Israel. The index ended with Vietnam. The United Arab Emirates stands 11 in the list of countries. But let's talk about the United Arab Emirates.

If you wish to visit UAE, specific regulations need to be followed along with particular documentation.

- If the UAE is your final destination, you must take a negative COVID-19 PCR test 96 hours before departure and bring the certificate to check.in. It includes passengers connecting to Dubai from specific destinations.
- The test should be taken a maximum of 96 hours before departure.
- The certificate must be for a polymerase chain reaction (PCR) test. Other test certificates, including antibody tests and home testing kits, are not accepted in Dubai.
- Bring an official, printed certificate in English or Arabic to check-in. SMS and digital certificates

are not accepted. A printed test certificate is a compulsion to board the flight.

These tests are an exception for children under the age of 12, and passengers who have a moderate or severe disability are exempt from this test. Every country has its regulations even after entering the country. In UAE, you must have masks on your face all the time. We'll then give you a complimentary travel hygiene kit containing gloves, a face mask, antibacterial wipes and a hand sanitizer. No one can touch each other; the crew members also have a full protective over: the court, masks, gloves and face screens. Once on a flight, a rapid antigen test, along with a temperature test, is given to everyone. Every room in every hotel is sanitized every day.

Lounge services have been modified to maintain strict hygiene levels and to reduce contact. Everyone in the lounge must wear a face mask, except while eating or drinking. Only the business class lounge is open, and other lounges are closed for the time being. There are spaced floor markers at the entrance to maintain social distancing and have reduced the number of people entering the lounge. Chairs and tables are spaced farther apart and are sanitized thoroughly after each use. Cleaning teams sanitize the washrooms after each use and frequently sanitize common touch-points. In showers, they provide hygienically packed towels and mats. They also have a Timeless Spa at Dubai International Airport Hotel, where a complimentary 15-minute treatment is available if you are eligible.

All the recliner seats in the quiet areas are sanitized after each use. The blankets and pillows are removed, and the newspapers and magazines are removed too. They offer some business services; however, our shoeshine service and children's area remain closed until further notice.

Several precautions are taken to maintain social distancing at the boarding gate, like standing on stickers to maintain a safe distance. Employees at the airport wear full personal protective equipment (PPE). Boarding gates and areas are deep-cleaned once everyone is on the plane. The cabin air is continuously cleaned with advanced HEPA air filters as powerful as those used in hospitals. Lavatories are frequently disinfected, and if the flight is longer than 1 hour and 30 minutes, then an extra crew member is added to clean the lavatories delicately. Before each flight, all aircraft undergo an improved cleaning and disinfection method. As a result, the UAE has also handled economic crises amid law and order, rather than being the most stable country during the pandemic.

So far, the UAE has provided more than 348 metric tonnes of aid to over 34 countries, supporting nearly 3,48,000 medical professionals in the process. They have put in a total of DH 116 million to combat the virus. On March 14, the UAE central bank announced that they are pumping in DH 100 billion, and the UAE cabinet approved 16 billion. Duty was suspended from all tolls until late 2020, and loans were given to small and medium-sized businesses to boost their operations after the pandemic.

Many other changes to the market include:

- No annual registration fees for commercial vehicles
- No toll gate for all vehicles
- No individual commercial real-estate registration fees
- 5 Bn for subsidies for water and electricity for both commercial and individual use
- Performance guarantees for projects up to AED 50 million waved for the startups
- All the bid bonds were suspended
- Industrial land leasing fees were reduced by 25 per cent
- Industrial and commercial penalties were waived
- Payment of approved government invoice within 15 days
- Up to 20 per cent rebate on rentals for the restaurant's tourism and entertainment sectors
- Tourism and municipality fees for the tourism and the entertainment sector are suspended for this year

100 per cent of government employees worked from home, and 80 per cent of private-sector employees worked from home. The UAE might not just be the safest place to visit in this pandemic but also one of the most stable countries. What is the most economically sound country?

FINANCIALLY MOST STABLE COUNTRY

The Economic Times conducted a study on the factors that define the economic stability of a country. Due to this pandemic, many countries had to suffer from financial crises. The lockdown imposed by the states and restrictions over international trade has crashed the economy for many countries. As per the factors, the most stable countries' list starts with Switzerland and Canada. It is followed by Australia being on the 10th. The economy of Switzerland proved to be one of the world's most stable economies for many reasons. Its long-term monetary security and political stability have made Switzerland a haven for investors, creating an increasingly dependent economy on a steady influx of foreign investment. They have also offered to provide liquidity for companies, prevent redundancies as much as possible and cover employee earnings loss.

Switzerland is responding quickly and effectively to the latest challenges through its international cooperation. It has taken many measures to alleviate the pandemic's economic and social effects, and it has so far contributed CHF 101.42 million to the global response to COVID-19. On 29 April 2020, the Federal Council has decided that Switzerland will provide CHF 400 million to support international relief in connection with COVID-19, especially for developing countries.

COVID-19 pandemic has a drastic effect on developing countries. They do not have a functioning health care system; their population does not have proper savings, regulated work conditions, or for that matter, stable work or social security to protect them against the loss of their livelihood. Malnutrition, HIV and tuberculosis also make many people in these countries more susceptible to this new lung disease. On top of all of it, they have small homes that make social distancing more challenging to follow, leading to the country's loss.

Switzerland is one of the countries that provided fast and unbureaucratic responses for countries suffering from COVID-19 to control the virus's spread. They helped other countries with humanitarian aid, including health care and food supplies, and bilateral development aid, which mitigates the social and economic impact and responds to global challenges by supporting other countries. The United Nations, the International Committee of the Red Cross (ICRC), the International Federation of Red Cross and Red Crescent Societies (IFRC), the G20 and other organizations made an appeal for financial support at the end of March, intending to maintain their operations during the crisis. Combined all together, they have offered to provide $5 trillion. These contributions are essential to deal with the current emergency, but they will further burden in increasingly unsustainable public debt in many countries. As a first step, the Federal Council wants Switzerland to grant the ICRC an interest-free loan of up to CHF 200 million, repayable within seven years.

Switzerland has already provided the World Health Organization (WHO) with CHF 3,00,000 to prepare hospitals for the pandemic at the beginning of

February 2020. Local organizations and health care units are training health care staff to treat COVID-19. On 2 April 2020, all UN member states except five countries signed a UN resolution to strengthen global solidarity connected with the COVID-19 pandemic. Switzerland was one of the key countries behind the initiative to work together and overcome the crises.

Swiss Humanitarian Aid (SHA) is also supplying equipment to China, Nepal, Serbia and Greece. It sent 10,000 protective suits to Italy on 8 April. Meanwhile, Switzerland's supply of material to combat the pandemic remains secure. Swiss NGO's are also adapting to the latest situation. They have also received funding from the Swiss Agency for Development and Cooperation (SDC).

Like many other countries, instead of firing the employees, Switzerland decided to reduce working hours for a certain period and cover part of the wages. It helped the employees to keep their families running, and the company sustained. Thanks to this regulation, employers hold on to already trained employees who can quickly resume activities. For their part, employees don't end up unemployed and keep their social protection intact. In comparison, in the United States, some 10 million workers have found themselves jobless in just three weeks.

There are many laws designed to secure the financial structure of the country. If the coronavirus drains the country's financial resources, the Swiss National Bank (SNB) could intervene with massive money injections. It was primarily the SNB that saved the largest Swiss bank (UBS) in 2008. The pressure on the central bank, which posted a profit of CHF 50 billion last year, would become quite strong in the event of significant social imbalances.

How will this pandemic affect an individual, a state or an atmosphere when the lives of the people living in this country are so drastically affected? Let me take you to my next chapter, “The Effects.”

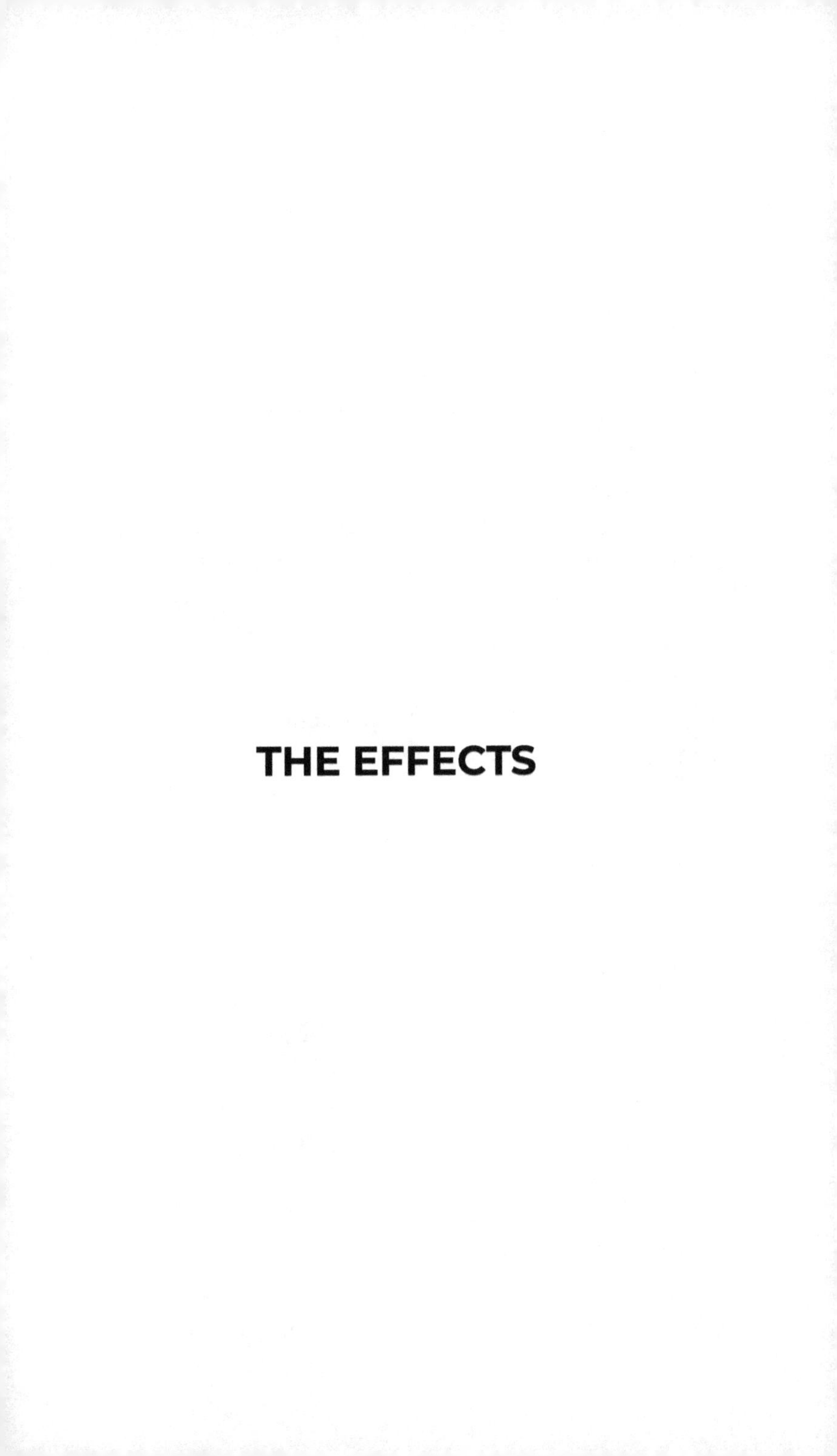

THE EFFECTS

The pandemic might stay for a couple of months, but the pandemic strains and the consequences might stay back for a long time. COVID-19 has affected people's lives so much that it has disrupted the global economy. It is estimated that, on average, it will take about a decade back to the state of the global economy that was in 2019. COVID-19 has rapidly affected our day-to-day lives and businesses. It has disrupted world trade and movements. Identifying the disease at an early stage is vital to control the virus's spread because it rapidly spreads from person to person. The effects of the pandemic can be classified into the following types:

- Environmental
- Healthcare
- Economical
- Social

Let's look over each aspect of the effects.

Environmental: This is one of the factors that can be said that it has done some good for people. There are various factors that influence the environment. COVID-19 has numerous effects on the environment and the climate. After the industrial revolution until 2020, an increasing amount of Greenhouse gas was released, which in turn increased the global temperatures, which melted the glaciers and raised the sea levels. Human activity causes environmental degradation and anthropogenic impact.

The global reduction in human activities like a ban on worldwide transportation, which includes the trades, has caused a major reduction in carbon emission, which leads to a reduction in global temperatures. China alone was accountable for reducing carbon emissions by 25 per cent and nitrogen emissions by 50 per cent. It is estimated that it saved a total of 77,000 lives in just two months.

Before the pandemic, researchers argued that reduced economic activity would help in flourishing the environment. As always, it was heard but was not acted upon. Due to this pandemic, many factories, ships and aeroplanes were seized, which restored a part of the environment. Reducing air pollution reduces the risk of both climatic change and COVID-19. However, it has not yet been fully defined what type of air pollution contributes to both air pollution and COVID-19. The Centre for Research on Energy and Clean Air reported that methods to contain the spreads of COVID-19 like lockdown and quarantine, resulted in a reduction in carbon emissions by 25 per cent, especially in Wuhan, China, where nitrogen dioxide levels dropped to 25-40 per cent. In 2019, China produced approximately 200 million fewer metric tonnes of carbon dioxide. This drop in nitrogen dioxide levels in China did not achieve the air quality of the standard that is considered acceptable by health authorities. Pollutants such as aerosol remained in the air.

A study conducted by global carbon emissions during the lockdown measured a 17 per cent decline in the carbon emission, and it is estimated that the total carbon emission might be reduced by 7 per cent by the end of the year globally. This is the biggest drop in carbon emissions since World War 2. However, the rebounding of companies might replenish the same carbon levels. There might not be a substantial decrease in carbon emission, but due to work from home strategies, there might be some amount of decrease in carbon emission. This might save a lot of fuel and time and give some mental peace. It is also estimated that there will be a decline in the demand for fossil fuel by 2 per cent. Since the beginning of the pandemic, the global need for fossil fuels has been reduced by 10 per cent.

In a study published in August 2020, there was a global decrease in NO emissions by 30 per cent by April and a 20 per cent reduction in SO2 emissions that weakens the cooling effect of the earth. This effect might not be much, but it is estimated to cool the earth by 0.01 to 0.005°C. Compared to the baseline scenario could avoid future warming by 0.3°C by 2050.

Certain people argued that this reduction came at the cost of drop-in economic development, and China might attempt to return to the previous rate of growth; they might ramp up the production, which will disrupt the energy market, in turn, worsening the conditions. The joint research team was led by the U.S. and China and have estimated that there was a decrease in 50 per cent of nitrogen dioxide emissions in East China, which is Wuhan then compared to earlier January. Post the lockdown, when some of the businesses were open for emissions, increased to 26 per cent in the initial days of February.

The Peruvian jungle experienced 14 oil spills from the beginning of the pandemic through early October 2020. Out of which, eight spills were in a single sector of Frontera Energy del Perú S.A. The primary reason for these spills was poor maintenance of the wells. As the businesses ceased to work, the wells were not maintained, which caused the oil spills. These oils seep into the ground, contaminating the groundwater and causing health issues.

In Venice, Italy, the water in the channels cleared, experiencing a greater water flow, and the sediments settled down, which are usually disrupted by boat traffic. All of this happened just after the lockdown was imposed at the beginning of March 2020. There was also a decrease in air pollution along the canals.

Due to the pandemic, fishing fleets would just sit idle, as there is no demand for the fish, which reduced the price of the fish. Some researchers estimate that the biomass of certain fish will double due to a sharp decrease in the fishing cycle. As of April 2020, signs of aquatic recovery remain mostly anecdotal. Some animals were also spotted more than usual; sea turtles were seen laying eggs on the beach due to lowered levels of human interference and light pollution. In the United States alone, fatal vehicle collisions with animals such as deer, elk, moose, bears and mountain lions fell by 58 per cent between March and April.

In Africa, there was a surge in bushmeat poaching. It is estimated that this surge is because the locals did not have any other alternative for income; there was also an increasing number of poaching for high-value products like ivory and Rhyno horn. In June 2020, Myanmar allowed the breeding of endangered animals such as tigers, pangolins and elephants. The Gabonese Republic decided to ban human consumption of bats and pangolins from stemming from the spread of zoonotic diseases. Other than high-value products, this pandemic also provided cover for illegal deforestation. Satellite imagery showed deforestation of the Amazon Rainforest surging by over 50 per cent compared to baseline levels. Due to rising unemployment, Pakistani labourers were recruited to plant 10 billion trees, which was the estimated net global loss of five years.

Due to the lockdown imposed, there was a surge in online deliveries. Many farmers and retail stores started putting all their products online where the consumers can come and purchase their goods, and it will be directly delivered at their doorsteps rather than driving and purchasing the goods from the stores or warehouses during the lockdown. This also helps the local farmers to sell their produce directly to the local people. This keeps a steady flow of income and helps consumers get organic supplies. Due to the fall of the meat industry, methane emissions from livestock continued to rise. Methane is a more potent Greenhouse gas than carbon dioxide.

Single-use medical materials have increased drastically due to this pandemic. Hospitals, airports and others had to use PPE kits every day, and all the used

PPE were single-use and cannot be recycled. This added a worldwide burden to the plastic pile up which adds up to the pile of plastic in nature that existed well before the pandemic. That pile will be piling up until the pandemic is over.

Energy and climate expert Constantine Samaras states that "a pandemic is the worst possible way to reduce emissions" and that "technological, behavioural and structural change is the best and only way to reduce emissions."

Healthcare: The COVID-19 pandemic has put some health systems under immense pressure and stretched others beyond their capacity. Responding to public health emergencies to minimize the loss requires a lot of resources, which included health care personnel. In fragile and conflict-affected countries, acts of violence during the COVID-19 pandemic, which include physiological threat, physical assault, individual weapons and elevation of homes, are some of the common forms of assaults during the COVID-19. The survey, which was completed in 155 countries over three weeks in May, confirmed that the impact was global but that low-income countries were most affected. The survey said that many people who needed treatment for cancer, diabetes, cardiovascular disease and other diseases did not get any treatment. Countries must ensure that they provide and balance treatment requirements for all patients.

Surveys say that the functioning of the hospitals in many countries are partially or completely disrupted. 53 per cent of the companies surveyed that their operations were partially or completely disrupted in many countries. Hospitals were unable to offer better service or treatment for 49 per cent diabetes-related patients, 42 per cent for cancer patients and 31 per cent for cardiovascular emergencies. Many hospitals had to adapt to the latest changes made by the country's regulations due to the pandemic. The hospitals needed to have the availability of ventilators along with ICU's to take care of the serious patients, along with dedicated nurses, to take care of the COVID-19 patients. To further adapt to the situation, the nurses had to be trained over the situation and the emergency protocol. They also had to train on treating patients and handling them appropriately to avoid further spreading of the virus.

Rehabilitation services have been disrupted in almost two-thirds, which is 63 per cent of countries. In the majority of the countries, all nurses were part of fully assigned to the COVID-19 patients. All screening programmes, like cancer treatments or tests, were all postponed for further notice. The major reason was that the patient was more susceptible to COVID-19, and if in case they attract COVID-19, it will be a potential loss for the patient and can be fatal. But the most common reasons for discontinuing or reducing services were cancellations of planned treatments, a decrease in public transport available and a lack of staff because health workers had been reassigned to support COVID-19 services. In one in five countries (20 per cent) reporting disruptions, one of the reasons for discontinuing services was a shortage of medicines, diagnostics and other technologies.

Globally, 2/3 of the countries have included NCD services in their national COVID-19 responses. It includes 72 per cent of high-income countries and 28 per cent of low-income countries. 17 per cent of the countries have started to allocate additional funds from the government budget to be included in the provision of NCD. Due to the growing economic crises in health care, many countries started to advise countries over the telephone for doctor consultation. This reduced the in-person consultation, which requires transportation, which can be risky and might not be possible in certain conditions. Globally, 58 per cent used telemedicine, also called expert doctor advice over the phone, in developed countries and 42 per cent in low-income countries.

In India, due to the lack of medical facilities, all the mild cases are asked to stay home quarantined until it gets cured or the condition deteriorates. All basic medication is provided by the hospitals and can be picked up from the hospital. Regular temperature checks and pulse rates are checked at home. If in case the condition deteriorates, the hospital can be called previously before arriving for further assistance and can be driven to the hospital. This exposes the family to infection, and the family has to take proper precautions to make sure they don't contract the infection.

Some of the major challenges faced by health care facilities are:

- Challenges faced in diagnostic and treatment of confirmed and unconfirmed cases.

- The burden increased on the medical institute and health care professionals to adapt and cure.
- Patients with other diseases and health problems are neglected.
- Health care professionals are at high risk.
- Medical chain supplies get disrupted as there is a sudden surge for the products.
- There are overloading of medical shops.
- There are requirements for health care equipment and training to adapt to the new environment.

Non-communicable diseases kill 41 million people each year, equivalent to 71 per cent of all deaths globally. Each year, 15 million people die from an NCD between the ages of 30 and 69 years; more than 85 per cent of these "premature" deaths occur in low-income and middle-income countries.

Economical: The COVID-19 pandemic has spread with towering speed spreading the infection and infecting millions, and bringing the global economy to a near standstill as the countries imposed lockdown and restrictions over international travelling. The medical expenses incurred by the countries drove the companies into a more economic loss. COVID-19 has triggered the deepest global recession in decades. It is known as the deepest global recession since 1945 to 1946. Among the 14 global recessions, this recession is known as the fourth deepest recession after 1914, 1930-32 and 1945-46 episodes. While the outcome is still uncertain, the pandemic will result in contractions across the vast majority of emerging markets and developing economies. It will also do lasting damage to labour productivity and potential output. The immediate policy priorities are to alleviate the human costs and attenuate near-term economic losses. The increase in global GDP in 1975 was 1.1; in 1982, it was 0.4; in 1991, it was 1.3; in 2009, it was -1.8, and in 2020 it was noted to be. Global GDP has drooped by 5.2 per cent. Certain economies show that the average growth in GDP has been -0.8 since 1975.

The COVID-19 recession is unique as it is the only such episode, at least since 1870, to have been triggered solely by a pandemic and the actions taken to contain it. The prolonged global recession of 1917-21 was partly driven by the Spanish flu pandemic during 1918-20 and also stemmed from the conclusion and aftermath of World War I. In 2009, the Swine flu pandemic was not a contributory factor to the global recession triggered by the financial crisis.

In Japan, preventive measures were able to slow the spread of the virus but triggered a fall in economic activity, magnifying acute adverse spillovers via trade and financial channels. As the Tokyo 2020 summer Olympics had to be postponed, it had compounded the adverse economic effects of the pandemic.

The spread of the pandemic has essentially stooped international travel and disrupted global economic chains, resulting in sharp changes in global trade. Flight to safety has triggered sharp falls in global equity markets, unprecedented capital outflows from Emerging Markets and Developing Economies (EMDEs), rising credit-risk spreads, and depreciation for many EMDE currencies.

Falling demand has decreased the price of the commodity, with a particularly substantial decrease in oil prices. As the pandemic spreads, measures to control the outbreak have limited or delayed the supply of critical inputs like automotive and electronics, along with stricter border controls and production delays that have all waited on trade.

The commodity market also had a major hit on the market. The price of oil declined by 50 per cent, coal by 25 per cent, natural gas by 26.8 per cent, natural rubber by 21.9 per cent, etc.; a known increase in the price of the commodity was gold. The price increased by 9.9 per cent. The drastic reduction in demand and prices for oil and industrial metals is a major headwind for commodity exporters, as commodities accounted for more than 75 per cent of exports in 2019 in the average member of this group. The investment in the extraction has drastically decreased due to which the government has suffered enormous losses, especially the countries that depend on commodity exports. Heightened investor risk aversion has tightened financial conditions for the few Low-Income Countries (LICs) that have borrowed from international capital markets, while contractions in major economies have reduced remittance flows, an important source of foreign funding in several LICs.

In addition, commodity exporters are struggling with domestic outbreaks and the side effects of mitigation measures. The number of these measures was initially higher in commodity exporters than in commodity importers, in part reflecting greater fears about the consequences of domestic outbreaks in countries where the capacity of the public health system is low.

Even before the COVID-19 pandemic hit, almost one-fifth of the low-income countries (LIC's) population was already experiencing an acute food insecurity crisis. The pandemic has further increased food insecurity in many LICs, including disruptions to imports and the effect of mitigation measures on supply chains and distribution networks. These disruptions may also lead to food price spikes that further erode the incomes of the poor, with evidence that prices of certain staples have already risen. Food insecurity could also be prolonged by the lack of access to critical inputs such as seeds and fertilizer, which could weigh on upcoming harvests. Many developed countries came forward to help under-developed and developing countries financially. But this also stands as a burden for the developing and mostly for under-developed countries. This stands as an extra expense to be collected from the taxpayers and paid back. This can develop the countries or get them in debt that can potentially explode the financial expenses.

Growth in LICs slowed sharply in the first half of 2020. The COVID-19 pandemic has spread to almost all LICs, and domestic mitigation measures have severely disrupted activity. Spillovers from recessions in significant economies have added to the problem, particularly in those LICs with strong trade linkages to China and the Euro Area. According to the average LIC, commodities account for two-thirds of goods exports, and the decrease in world markets has weighed heavily on industrial commodity exporters.

In short, this pandemic has led to:

- Slowing of manufacturing and trading of goods
- Poor cash flow in the market
- Revenue growth came almost to a halt
- Loss in international business
- High debt on the countries that have acquired loans
- Disrupted the trade chain business

The question arises, will we ever get out of this economic loss?

The sharp fall in activity in the first half of this year has contributed to a decline in global trade of about 13.4 per cent in 2020. A gradual recovery is expected to begin in the second half of the year as sanctions are removed, travel returns to more normal levels and factories restore inventories. Historically, this rebound is supposed to be slow. However, representing the extraordinary existence of the current situation, it will take time to regain trust, replace distressed companies and create virus-safe working and entertainment environments. In particular, utilities do not benefit as much as production when inventories are restored and when sales of durables take place following a time of deferral. Owing to stricter border protection procedures, it will take longer for air traffic to return to the standards of the industry in recent years. Above all, decreased number of passengers would raise the price of air travel. The current global recession is predicted to last just one year; in other words, the growth rate of global GDP per capita is estimated to turn positive in 2021.

Social: The COVID-19 pandemic has far-reaching consequences beyond the transmission of the disease itself and the quarantine effort, including its political, cultural and social influence. Many regional leaders of the Communist Party of China (CPC) have been dismissed for poor handling of the quarantine situation in Central China. Some analysts suggest that it was likely to shield Communist Party Secretary-General Xi Jinping from people's indignation at the coronavirus pandemic. Protests in the social administration regions of Hong Kong have intensified due to concerns of immigrants from mainland China. Taiwan also raised questions about the inclusion of the People's Republic of China travel ban as part of the "One-China Principle" and its contested political status.

Many countries used the outbreak to show support towards China. Colombian Prime Minister Hun Sen made a special visit to China intending to show support towards China from Colombia. The treasurer of Australia was also unable to keep up with the finances due to the pandemic outbreak. The United States President Donald Trump was criticized for his response over the pandemic. He was also accused of making several misleading claims, like providing adequate information about the pandemic, providing false claims and down-paying the pandemic significance. He was also claimed for closing down the global health security unit of the United States National Security Council, which was specifically made for a potential pandemic.

The government of the Islamic Republic of Iran was highly affected by the virus. At least two dozen employees of the Iranian legislature, along with 15 other top government officers, which include their vice-president, contracted COVID-19. Iran, Jordan, Morocco, Oman and Yemen banned the printing and distribution of newspapers as it might expedite the spreading of the virus. This change in the process leads to the development of the digital newspaper.

The educational system has also been affected worldwide due to the closure of schools and universities. As per the data released by UNESCO on 25 March, 165 countries were affected worldwide, which affected 1.5 billion students worldwide, which accounted for about 87 per cent of the students. The education system has been accounted for the most changes in the century. To adapt to the latest situation due to the pandemic, schools and universities have started online classes. With the further advancement of the pandemic, many schools have also started online exams. This is termed as the new future of distance learning.

Coronavirus is also known to be unequal. Pandemic state and less availability of medical resources increased the cost of the treatment. If a person from a low-income family is infected, they might not have the resources to finance the cure. Industrial employees and hard labour did not have their jobs due to the lockdown, which further increased the financial insecurities, which reduced or, in some cases, depleted the financial resources of the individual. On the other hand, many people have adopted for work from home. Employees working from home mostly saved their money since they did not have to travel and had more time to cook their food. One of the major benefits of work-from-home employees had families migrated to live closer, which saved rents or, in some cases, migrated to lower-cost communities. This created inequality among the employees working from home and employees who did not have jobs. In other words, it can be defined as "rich became richer and poor became poor."

Hypotheses on why this is the case include the fact that disadvantaged households are more likely to live in cramped accommodation and work in low-level occupations, such as supermarkets and elderly care, which are considered necessary during the recession. In the United States, millions of low-income individuals may lack access to health insurance because they are uninsured or under-insured. The rise in unemployment has led to a financial downturn compounded by social isolation due to quarantine and social-distancing guidelines. Combined with fear and anxiety have led to a potential increase in suicides. Chaos and the detrimental consequences of the COVID-19 pandemic may have triggered a disastrous future. It can also have the opposite impact by concentrating on the more imminent danger of a pandemic rather than on the global crisis or on the mitigation of other disasters. The risk factor has also accelerated crime rates around the world, especially in low-economic countries, which have made the place unsafe for life in most regions. Many countries have registered a growing amount of domestic sailing and intimate partner sailing. Financial vulnerability, tension and confusion have also contributed to escalated assaults at home, with abusers able to monitor vast numbers of their victims' everyday lives. The United Nations Secretary-General António Guterres called for an end to domestic violence.

Mandatory stays at home during the lockdown had a major impact on personal gathering. Festivals and events were replaced by teleconferencing calls. Some unconventional method was used to maintain social distancing like balcony sing-along for a concert of a birthday party. Replacement of gathering had a significant effect on mental health during the crisis. Due to the imposement of the lockdown, it is important that we keep a close watch on our loved ones and keep a tab on their mental state and health status; in the normal situation going out clears the mind and helps us feel refreshed, which feels like positive energy. With no one to talk to or clear their minds, they might go into depression.

One of the major unseen factors that affect society is rumours. There was a forward message spreading on WhatsApp that "A person with mild fever, cold and cough went to a hospital to get himself checked. He was declared corona-positive and forcefully admitted to the hospital. A few days later, he suddenly passed away. All arrangements were made to cremate the body. But on the pressure of family members, the body was shown to them, and several of his body parts were found missing." Noticing the situation, Mumbai police panicked. It was being said that even people who were not infected by COVID-19 were being declared positive. Such people were forcefully admitted to hospitals and their vital organs extracted. It was said that the case was reported from the Gorai area of northwest Mumbai.

A team was set up to have a report created on the case. The final report concluded that it was fake news, and the pictures shared with the post were from Lucknow. Upon locating the loop of the post, it was identified that the post was under circulation before COVID-19. Initially, the post was shared as an outcome of organ trafficking in Mumbai; later, it was modified as per the situation. After reading a fact check from the Aaj Tak, it was concluded that Versha Verma, a Lucknow-based social worker, filed an FIR against "Delhi Crime Press." Versha runs an NGO in Lucknow, which performs the last rites of unclaimed bodies. The pictures used in the viral post were taken from Versha's Facebook page. The body seen in the pictures belonged to a woman who was severely ill and died in a government hospital in Lucknow.

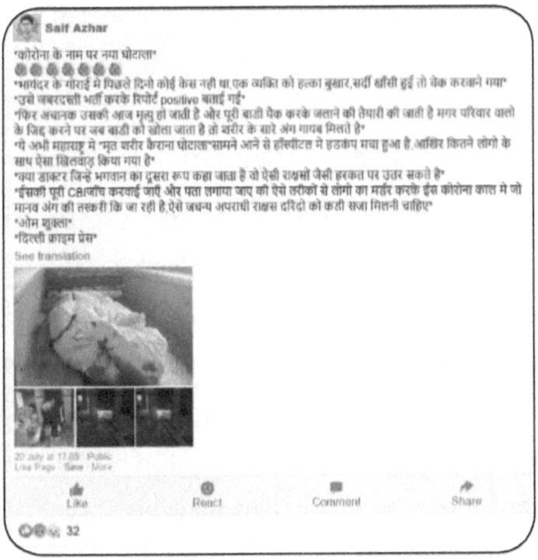

The language used in the text is Hindi.

Concerning the situation, I asked Shirin how the hospital looks at a subject like this. If a patient dies of COVID-19, all laboratory results and vitals have to be readily recorded for examination, and the hospital notifies the concerned authorities. Since the body cannot be sent out or returned. The body must be cremated inside the institution or the nearest criminology clinic. Before the cremation, a police detective checks and verifies the records for possible criminal conduct. Once the records are reviewed, the officer will accompany them to the cremation area. The bodies are criminated in front of the officer. If the documents are not checked, then the hospital must explain the cause. If any wrongdoings have been identified, then necessary action will be taken against the hospital.

Many hospitals that had permission to release the body for religious purposes had to disinfect the body and seal it in a box. Christians have a tradition of burying their dead. Hospitals had to pack the body in an airtight glass box so that the box's air does not leak out and is passed on to the relevant authorities.

It is not just with India. It has been happening all over the world. Due to work from home policies and many people losing their time, most people have spent most of their time scrolling feeds over social media, which stood as a significant factor for the rumours to spread like wildfire. In many cases, people have been scrolling their feeds to know more about the situation and get false information. It is not that no wrong things are happening worldwide, but the most crucial factor is a fact check. If a fact check is not possible, then the information should not be shared with others. There can be instances where the hospital and the police officers are working together to smuggle organs, but it should not affect all the neighbourhood hospitals. With a rise in concerns due to the pandemic, the last thing this world needs is chaos.

Living in this time, everyone feels like when will the old times return. When will all of this end? Let me take you to my next chapter, "The End."

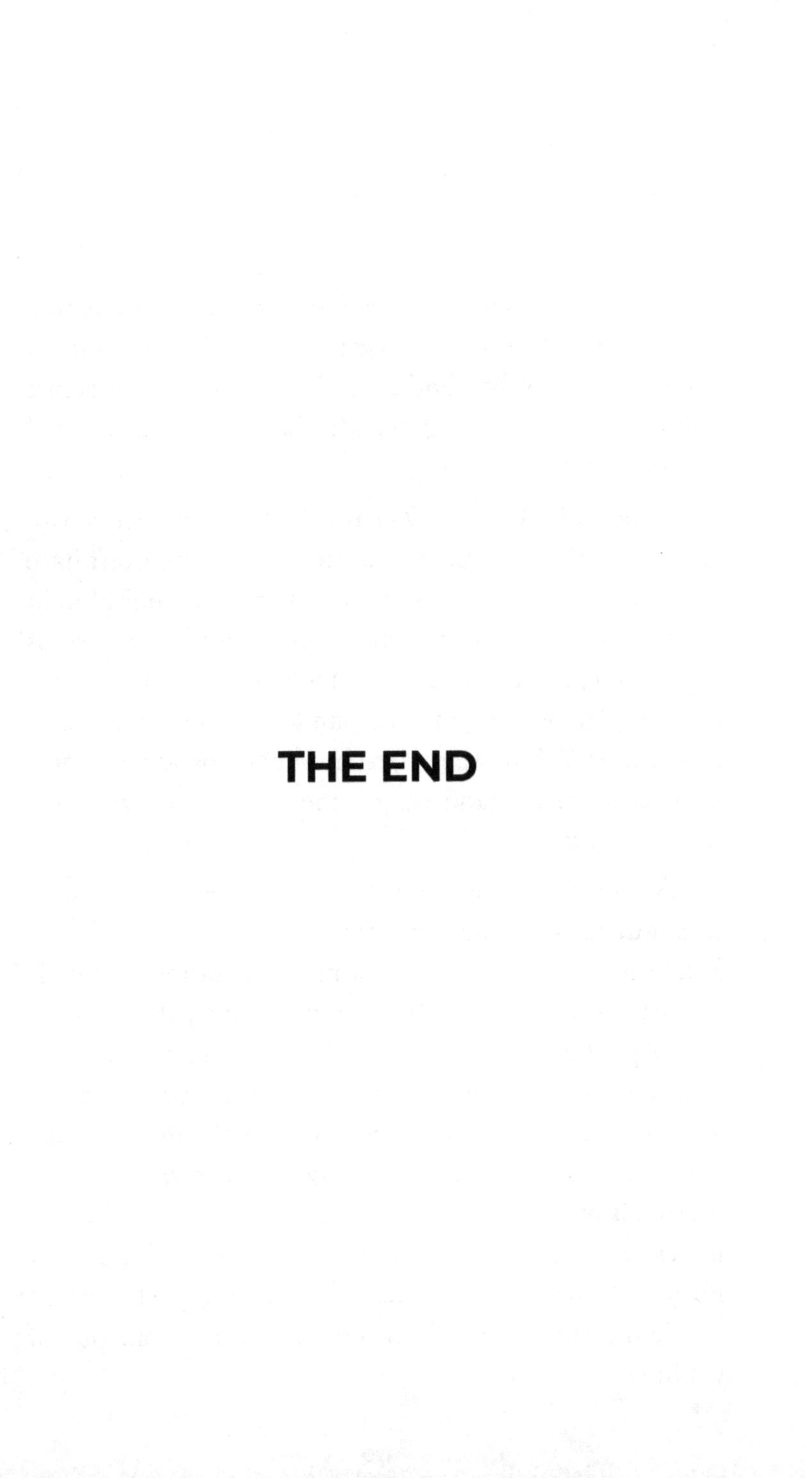

THE END

All that begins needs to have an end; so do pandemics. Yet, we do not have a cure or antidote to help us bring an end to the pandemic. So, how is the pandemic going to end? Is it going to end? Have we ever eradicated any such sort of disease?

Expert of COVID-19 claims that this pandemic will stop when there is a cure or a vaccine. Yet, we don't have a cure or a vaccine. So, isn't it coming to an end? Should we have to live the same way we live now? The answer is a good one, but there's a catch. How do we know that we are completely free from the pandemic, and it is safe to go outside? Before we understand how a pandemic ends, we need to understand what it means. How do we know that it's over?

According to medical historians, there are two forms of pandemic's ending: a medical end and a societal end. When nobody left to get ill, a medical ending occurs. It doesn't mean that everybody is dead, even if that's one way a pandemic will stop. While the infection may no longer propagate, an epidemic may effectively come to an end, either because many individuals are immune, have been vaccinated or simply because of stringent social distancing policies that render it difficult for the infection to attract new victims. The fearful Bubonic Plague is the best example of a medically eliminated pandemic since it has been eradicated as it ran out of victims.

Bubonic Plague is one of the three forms of infection caused by Yersinia pestis. Flu-like symptoms develop one to seven days after exposure to the bacteria. These symptoms include fever, exhaustion and vomiting. Swollen and swollen lymph nodes are formed in the area adjacent to where the bacteria have infected the skin. During the Bubonic Plague, quarantine steps were implemented to keep the sick from exiting the house unless they were absolutely necessary. The Black Plague that occurred in 1346-1353 also came to an end with the introduction of quarantine. The Spanish flu, which happened in 1918, also ended when those affected died or became immune. At the moment, no one knew how the epidemic spread, but they were confident it would spread in the vicinity. So, they largely adopted a quarantine measure, and the required medicine was given to the sick. Experts are not sure precisely when any epidemic ended; it either ran out of victims, weakened by the cold weather or may have mutated to be less lethal.

Eventually, both of these outbreaks stopped, but the disease was not gone. Currently, it's still around now. It's just the approach that the pandemic will end medically. But the pandemic still has another end called the "social end." A social end to the pandemic does not mean that the epidemic is gone; it only means that people have learned to deal with it. The pandemic will end psychologically as people stop fearing the epidemic, become sick with quarantine limits and conclude that they can risk catching the virus and move on with their everyday lives. The Spanish flu is an excellent indicator of the socioeconomic end of the pandemic. The aggressive and deadly strain of the flu virus that tore across the globe and killed millions prompted one doctor to say that it "demonstrated the inferiority of human inventions in the destruction of human life."

That was a tough saying, given that the globe was one at the time of the eruption in the bloody trench wars of the world war. The strain gradually evolved into a less serious influenza version, and the medical pandemic steadily collapsed, even though the outbreak had not gone anywhere. Yet even though the epidemic began to wreak havoc, the pandemic stopped economically. At the end of World War One, people everywhere were sick of death and misery, and they were eager for a new start. Since the hardships of war, people were willing to risk sickness to return to normal life as quickly as possible. The truth is, this is not the case, either. Pandemics do not end medically and then socially, but they end socially until they end medically. It is almost unlikely to get a proper medical end. In most cases, we learn to deal with the disease and control its dissemination to avoid widespread spreads, but seldom is it a completely medically eradicated disease.

Smallpox is one of the only exceptions. It has been around for more than 3,000 years. 30 per cent of those who have contracted the mysterious disease have died a miserable death. In 1633, soon after the first European explorers arrived in the New World, a smallpox outbreak ravaged the local population. The epidemic was arriving with the adventurers. None of the native people had immunity from the disease. It spread like flames, killing up to 90-95 per cent of the native population in some of the hardest-hit areas. There are a few different ways in which our attempts to combat it have been so successful. The most notable breakthrough has been the discovery of an effective long-term vaccine. The disease's peculiar symptoms, the rash that develops into pus-filled patches that crust and then fall off, have made it possible to diagnose the disease, and affected individuals could be quarantined easily, restricting the spread of the disease.

Another aspect that helped defeat smallpox was that it could not be spread by wildlife. It means that once the disease was eradicated from humans, we no longer had to worry that it would continue to circulate and mutate in wildlife reemerging in the future. Both of these factors contributed to making it one of the only viruses that we can confidently claim to have been medically eradicated. The social aspect of a pandemic can be just as dangerous as the disease itself or even more so. Back during the Ebola outbreak in West Africa, the disease progresses quicker than the disease itself. We should prepare to fight the terror of ignorance as vigorously and thoughtfully as we fight against every other disease. In that situation, anxiety is liable to do terrible harm to vulnerable people, even places that have never had a single case of disease during an outbreak. The fear of each recent outbreak only exacerbates the fear of the next.

Because the next epidemic is imminent, we need to learn how to cope with the pandemic panic and minimize the epidemic's social damage. Pandemics are one of the significant challenges we humans face in modern times. The next pandemic is expected to cost over $60 billion and kill 30 million people in just six months. As the number of infectious diseases increases and people migrate more and more rapidly than ever before, the possibility of a big global pandemic continues to increase. It might sound intimidating, but don't think about it. I have a roadmap for how to minimize the effects of the next epidemic. Since most outbreaks originate in animals, better surveillance of disease outbreaks in animal species and better coordination and quick response to new diseases is expected to avoid further outbreaks and give countries time to prepare for the next. So, the question we began with is, when's the end of the COVID-19 pandemic?

It is clear that it will not stop medically, at least until we have a vaccine. It will then take years to vaccinate the entire planet and assume that the pandemic has ended medically even though we need to look out for new strains of the virus. Socially, though, it seems like this pandemic will quickly stop, regardless of whether it is medically secure or not. Citizens are becoming irritated with social distancing and quarantine, and the economic and social effects of months of closure are beginning to worry citizens rather than the virus itself. The conclusion of the pandemic will not be a sudden triumph. And if vaccines are made, it will take years for the whole world to be vaccinated. Before it occurs, the pandemic is expected to continue to stop economically, as populations and countries continue to relax their quarantine behaviour. Another aspect that makes it impossible to detect the end of a pandemic is that the disease has varying consequences in different regions.

Even as the disease progresses across the globe, some areas may see a severe epidemic and a high mortality rate as we have seen in Italy. In contrast, other regions may not have any cases at all. At some point, the World Health Organisation will announce the conclusion of the global pandemic emergency. However, particular countries may have already defeated them, although others may still be battling the outbreak. Whatever happens, we will need to continue to deal with the epidemic and control its spread while hoping for a medical end to the pandemic. Since the next pandemic could be right around the corner, it would be prudent to keep our quarantine and social distance skills sharp for the future. This pandemic is nowhere close to ending medically. So, until it ends medically, let's follow social distancing and minimum physical contact with outsiders. With the growing number of applications like Facetime, WhatsApp video calls, etc., we can keep in touch with our loved ones.

Due to this lockdown, my neighbour had made a habit of going to our terrace for fresh air. One day he saw a girl on the neighbourhood terrace. He liked the girl, so he sent a drone with his contact info on it. He started talking to her and finally fell in love. They are in a relationship now. Not everything has to be bad. They are waiting for everything to end, so they can go out together. It is just a perspective of seeing the good in everything. If the lockdown had not started, then he would not have found his first love. Many must have got in touch with their old friend or someone new or a person who never thought you would ever meet with much free time available. Well, that is life. Many must also have lost their loved ones due to COVID-19. If you are one of them, trust me, everything will be all right. If you feel low or have a concern, then talk to your friends or family because no matter what happens, life must go on.

Two years ago, I asked a question to myself, “What is the purpose of my life?” This pandemic has answered this question after I met a great friend. I am glad we met. So, what is the purpose of your life? Don’t worry; I have a new book coming very soon, “The Purpose.” I have answered many questions in this book, like why we are alive, or what is our purpose in our life and many other questions. If you liked this book, I am certain you will like “The Purpose.” It is not a philosophical book; it is a book that gives a scientific approach to life. Stay tuned for “The Purpose.”

ABOUT THE AUTHOR

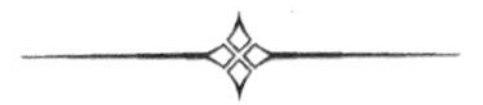

Hey, smart people! Good to see you in the end. Don't worry; it is not the end. I have another book waiting for you with some new scientific theories. By the way, my name is Harish Ankadala. I hope you learned a lot from this book. Knowledge should be accessible to everyone. Everyone has the right to know and understand. That is the reason I started writing this book. Scientific concepts are one of the things that not everyone understands. Well, it isn't straightforward, I must say that. I had to do a lot of research while writing this book. Not everyone has access to all the search papers that I went through and certainly didn't have the patience to understand them. Those numbers do piss me off. But I'm on a mission to make scientific ideas more accessible and understandable to everyone.

During the pandemic, I heard many people misinterpreting the situation. So, I came ahead with a book to clear all the confusion with scientific theories. I hope that you love this book and share it with your loved ones. If you have any questions, then please ask me, and I will be happy to answer them. You can ask them on my website or my Instagram the_introspective_mind1.

www.ingramcontent.com/pod-product-compliance
Lightning Source LLC
Chambersburg PA
CBHW051301250726
48656CB00004B/1410

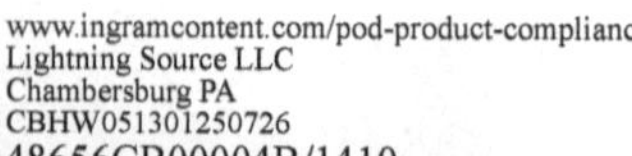